Advance p

Living Life as a

The Transformative Power of Daily Gratitude
by Nina Lesowitz and Mary Beth Sammons

"I have learned that the greatest joy and happiness comes from what we do to enrich other people's lives and our own spiritual lives. *Living Life as a Thank You* shows you how to connect with other people from a place of thankfulness, which in turn promotes greater harmony and happiness for all."

—Marla Maples, actress, television host,
and spiritual motivator

"*Living Life as a Thank You* is a healing guidebook for people looking to bring more gratitude—as well as more joy and stronger social connections—into their lives. It reminds us that life is not a rehearsal, but something to be celebrated and savored to the fullest. I am convinced that if readers take even one small gratitude practice from this book they will bring greater happiness into their lives while contributing to the greater good. Inspirational and spiritual, this book is a great how-to companion for people following the science of appreciation."

—Christine Carter, PhD, executive director of the
Greater Good Science Center at UC Berkeley and author of
Raising Happiness and *The Other Side of Silence*

"Twenty years ago, we gathered friends together to write about, talk about, and do Random Acts of Kindness, and from this small group a kindness movement was born that circled the globe. With *Living Life as a Thank You*, Nina and Mary Beth have tapped into something just as deep and powerful that can truly transform people's lives—our deep and abiding need to feel and live from a place of gratitude."

—Will Glennon, founder, The Random Acts of Kindness Foundation and author of *Practice Random Acts of Kindness*

"This book will put a smile on your face and a lift in your step, and give you plenty of reminders that saying 'thanks' costs nothing, but delivers a lot!"

—Jan Yanehiro, Emmy-winning broadcaster and author of *This is Not the Life I Ordered*

"Thank you, thank you, thank you for *Living Life as a Thank You*. I am grateful for the inspiring stories, the simple, clear exercises with profound results, and the empowering reminder that an attitude of gratitude boosts self-esteem, well-being, and appreciation for the precious gifts that fill our days. This is a must-read for everyone who desires peace and happiness."

—Susyn Reeve, author of *Choose Peace & Happiness*

"In our day and age, the daily practice of gratitude and acceptance is arguably the most important spiritual routine we should all embrace. Nina Lesowitz and Mary Beth Sammons found an entertaining and wonderful way to make it easy for us to live life as one big thank you!"

—Gahl Eden Sasson, author of *A Wish Can Change Your Life*

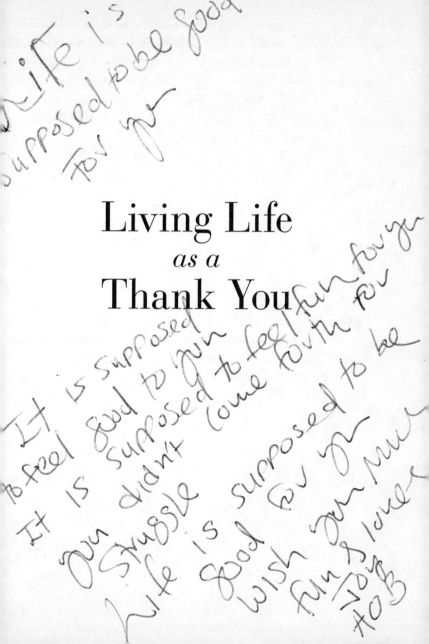

Living Life
as a
Thank You

Life is
supposed to be good
for you

It is supposed
to feel good to you
It is supposed to feel fun for you
you didn't come forth for
struggle
Life is supposed
good for you
wish you much
fun & love
xox

Living Life
as a
Thank You

The Transformative Power of
Daily Gratitude

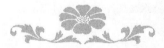

By Nina Lesowitz and Mary Beth Sammons

Published in the United States by Viva Editions, an imprint of Cleis Press Inc., P.O. Box 14697, San Francisco, California 94114.

Printed in Canada.
Cover design: Scott Idleman
Text design: Frank Wiedemann
10 9 8 7 6 5 4 3 2 1
ISBN: 978–1-57344–368–5

"Weather Report" copyright © 2009 by BJ Gallagher. Reprinted with permission of the author.

Library of Congress Cataloging-in-Publication Data

Lesowitz, Nina.
Living life as a thank you : the transformative power of gratitude in your life / by Nina Lesowitz and Mary Beth Sammons.
    p. cm.
Includes bibliographical references and index.
ISBN 978-1-57344-368-5 (trade paper : alk. paper)
1. Gratitude. 2. Conduct of life. 3. Quality of life. I. Sammons, Mary Beth. II. Title.
BF575.G68L47 2009
179'.9--dc22
                                    2009029140

To Martin, Mara, and Jaime, who give me lots of reasons to say thank you every day

—Nina Lesowitz

To Caitlin, Thomas, and Emily, who let me share my love daily, with gratitude

—Mary Beth Sammons

ACKNOWLEDGMENTS

Nina Lesowitz

Just as a journey begins with a single step, opening your heart to new possibilities begins with the seed of an idea. For me, the concept of gratitude was planted by Mary Jane Ryan's book *Attitudes of Gratitude*. I read the book over ten years ago and planned to return to it—one day—when I was ready to let go of my patterns and embrace a new way of being. Thank you, Mary Jane.

I am so grateful to everyone at Viva Editions, with a special place in my heart for Brenda Knight for her guidance and support. I am thankful every day for Mary Beth Sammons. Her entry into my life as a business partner, co-author, and friend was felicitous, and continues to feel like a daily miracle.

For some people, gratitude is an intrinsic part of their spirit. My late mother, Tomoko, was the embodiment of a grateful attitude; memories of her inspire me as I attempt to channel her natural ability to appreciate life's many simple and profound blessings. My husband, Martin, inspires me with his innate sense of gratitude, and I am eternally grateful to him for enhancing my life in so many ways.

To my children, Mara and Jaime: how did I get so lucky to be your mom? Once, I dreamed of having two daughters who would grow into women I would love to be friends with, and now, eighteen-plus years later, you are that and so very much more.

To all the researchers in the field of gratitude studies, thank you for enlightening us about the transformative power of thankfulness. To the individuals featured in this book, I am most appreciative. It is an honor to be able to share your stories. To my good friends and family, thank you for all that you bring to my life.

Mary Beth Sammons

"Be careful what you pray for" is a mantra I've been paying close attention to in recent years. When we launched this project to understand the power of gratitude in people's lives, I said a silent prayer that in the process I would learn more about how to manifest it in my own life. The universe responded promptly: I lost my job while taking care of my aging father, and then I lost him too. The worst recession in decades swooped in. My challenge had presented itself. I was determined not to bemoan the losses, but to embrace the light that could be found in the darkness.

It sounds corny, but the touch of adversity has propelled me to embrace the good in every moment. My father, Paul Von Driska, used to call it "finding a little Christmas in every day." I learned how to be grateful for simple pleasures. I learned to pay attention to the small moments, to the extraordinary people in my everyday life—and to practice saying thank you to those who joined me in my new landscape for living. I quickly realized we were on to something.

I am grateful first to Brenda Knight and Nina Lesowitz for the opportunity to see the difference thankfulness makes in daily living—not just in other's lives, but in my own. It is a wonderful experience to work with colleagues on a project one you feel passionately about, and even better to become friends in the process.

I am especially thankful for my three children—Caitlin, Thomas, and Emily—and the light they bring into my life. They keep me on the edge of my seat, and they have fulfilled my life dream to be a mom and to learn how much one can love.

I thank all my friends who stand by me and make me smile.

And I thank all those who shared their stories in this book to inspire others. You captured my heart, and I know you will bring joy and new hope into the lives of others. Thank you for sharing your lives with me.

TABLE OF CONTENTS

I've received so many wonderful e-mails and notes from folks who have read on the news that my husband, Bob, is back in Iraq and Afghanistan three years after his injury in Balad from a roadside bomb. So many people have been so supportive of his desire to go back in honor of those who have served, who are serving, and who have returned from the wars injured or different.

I've subconsciously waited for this day to come for almost two years now, once I realized Bob would recover enough to go back to the work he loves. I give thanks that he can pursue his dreams again.

During the last three years, a lot has changed in our family. I'd like to believe that the personal tragedy has transformed in time to a testament of the resilience of the human spirit—our spirits, and the souls of the thousands of people who have come into our lives as blessing. For this I am grateful.

I have decided to live life out of that place of gratitude. I won't live my life worrying that lightning will strike twice. I've already been reminded just how precious it is. As Bob says often to me, if I worry about safety or danger, "You could step off the curb in Manhattan and get hit by a bus." And he is right. Life is unpredictable. It's impossible to script. In fact it's perfectly imperfect.

I have been honored to meet so many individuals and families who are facing their own challenges that life has hurled at them.

It makes me think twice about the blessings that have come into our lives. They include: my children; family, faith, and friends. I'm also thankful for the chance to advocate on behalf of the brain-injured community and our wounded service members. The communities of those who have struggled or made a journey have taught me much. They've taught me about the ability to let go and understand we are not in control, and the ability to focus on the little things and sometimes go day by day. For this I am very grateful.

Through all this, I have learned about the power of

thankfulness. Those of you who are facing challenges in your lives will want to read about the power of staying thankful in difficult times. *Living Life as a Thank You* is a must-read for discovering how gratitude can create happiness in our lives.

The book serves as a guide for bringing to our awareness the things for which we can still be grateful, and this helps evoke joy in the midst of uncertainty. The book also shows us, powerfully, that by giving thanks and giving to others out of that gratitude, we will feel as if we have more than we thought we did.

Gratitude isn't always easy to come by, especially in challenging times. *Living Life as a Thank You* offers some practical techniques to help us get in touch with the parent of all virtues—gratefulness. It is guaranteed to help you cultivate gratitude and be genuinely thankful.

Lee Woodruff

Lee Woodruff's career as a bestselling author was launched with In an Instant, *a memoir she co-wrote with her husband, journalist Bob Woodruff, after he suffered a nearly fatal head injury while embedded with troops in Iraq in 2006. Her second book, a collection of autobiographical essays called* Perfectly Imperfect: A Life in Progress, *delivers a collection of almost 20 essays about juggling life as a busy mom to four kids, a loving wife, a daughter of aging parents, a friend, and a real-life person who doesn't always have the answers. Contact Lee at* www.leewoodruff.com *or through the Bob Woodruff Foundation at* www.Remind.org.

INTRODUCTION

Imagine living as if each day were a gift. Imagine that everywhere you went people smiled and said, "Thank you," and you in turn were filled with joy and gratitude from the moment you woke up until you hit the pillow at night, your heart filled with joy, your mind still and calm. Just imagine, a world without grumbling, a world where everyone is happy and grateful for where they are.

Tired of walking around with a hole in your heart? Need more inspiration?

Studies show—and experts counsel—that gratitude is a key component for personal happiness. People who are grateful about specific things in their past, who celebrate the triumphs, instead of focusing on losses or bitter disappointments, tend to be more satisfied in the present. In the popular book *The Secret*, author Rhonda Byrne writes: "With all that I have read and all that I have experienced in my own life using the Secret, the power of gratitude stands above everything else. If you do only one thing with the knowledge of the book, use gratitude until it becomes your way of life."

Cultivating an attitude of gratitude goes beyond giving thanks on holidays or for gifts.

When we practice daily thankfulness, we have the potential to transform our reality. And when we give thanks for the unexpected good, we are setting a life energy in motion to produce all that is good.

The buzz about the power of gratitude is overwhelmingly positive. Jeffrey Zaslow, a columnist for the *Wall Street Journal*, recently wrote that there may be a positive byproduct of the troubled economic times that followed the 2008 stock market dive: a decrease in the urge to complain. "People who still have jobs are finding reasons to be appreciative. It feels unseemly to complain about not getting a raise when your neighbor is unemployed," he wrote. "Homeowners are unhappy that home values have fallen, but it's a relief to avoid foreclosure."

Indeed, in these times of economic woes, gratitude is popping up everywhere. Turn on the TV. We listened as a career coach on *The Today Show* advised job seekers to put the words "Thank you" in their job search tool kit, declaring that the key to distinguishing oneself from the masses is to send a thank-you note. Or click onto Facebook, the popular social networking site, and check out the gratitude groups, where hundreds of people log on each day to give thanks for everything from the sun rising that morning to their neighborhood dog park. Cathy, of Greenville, South Carolina, wrote: "I am grateful for a bark park to take my dog-children to, so I picked up extra poop and trash this morning." Mary, from Philadelphia, wrote: "I am so grateful for the beautiful snow outside."

Gratitude floats our boats and has us doing all kinds of things inspired by joy. Gratitude can help us transform our fears into courage, our anger into forgiveness, our isolation into belonging, and another's pain into healing. Saying "Thank you" every day will create feelings of love, compassion and hope.

Gratitude makes us healthier. Experts now tell us that giving thanks makes us happier and more resilient, and it strengthens our relationships and reduces our stress. When we give thanks, we feel more connected to the flow of life, and less alone in our struggles and fears. "To bless whatever there is, and for no other reason but simply because it is, that is what we are made for as human beings," David Steindl-Rast writes in *Gratefulness, the Heart of Prayer: An Approach to Life in Fullness.*

When gratitude rules, grumbles dissolve. Last spring, a Kansas City, Missouri, minister launched a nonprofit organization to put an end to complaining. Rev. Will Bowen created A Complaint Free World Inc., distributing almost 6 million purple bracelets emblazoned with the group's name. When wearers find themselves complaining, they're asked to switch bracelets to their other wrists. The goal is to go 21 days without having to switch.

Grateful for tough times? You betcha, says Rev. Bowen, who believes the bad economy may be just the catalyst we need to reevaluate our lives. "In good times, people often take for granted what they have, and whine about what they don't have," he says. "Bad times make people more grateful."

The fact is that the art of living—for that is what we speak about when we speak of gratitude—isn't something that comes naturally to most people. We need to work intentionally to increase the intensity, duration, and frequency of positive, grateful feelings.

In *Living Life as a Thank You: The Transformative Power of Gratitude in Your Life,* we have asked dozens of people to clue us in to the secret to cultivating gratitude in our lives. In addition to the inspiring stories of individuals who are focused on a strategy of thankfulness to bring about abundant living, we have also included practices throughout the book to help you get started, or to remind you to take the time to recognize the blessings in your life.

As guides to what we talk about as "great-full" living, we take you inside the hearts and minds of people who have tapped into the power of gratitude in their lives. Some came by their enlightenment through an epiphany moment, some through years of training, and others by pure serendipity.

We hope you'll be inspired by the incredible stories in this book. Sometimes, all it takes is one wise person to lead the way. If we listen closely to someone who has come back from the brink, we can learn from them. Without fail, those people teach us to appreciate what we currently take for granted.

We are grateful to the people who shared their stories in this book. They come from all walks of life with completely different stories to tell, yet they all managed to find some measure of happiness and peace in their lives.

In ancient Roman times, Cicero said, "Gratitude is not only the greatest of virtues, but the parent of all the others." Having an attitude of gratitude is not new advice, but in our fast-paced 21st-century lives, we need extra reminders to get in touch with the essence of life before our lives fast-forward to our final days.

With great-fullness,
Nina and Mary Beth

CHAPTER ONE
THANK-YOU POWER:
STAY WELL

Don't be concerned about being disloyal to your
pain by being joyous.

—Pir Vilayat Inayat Khan

We are living in groundbreaking, defining times, when
most of us find ourselves uncertain about how we are
going to navigate what lies ahead.

However, the promise of the new is on the horizon,
making this an ideal time to reevaluate how we envision
our lives and the spirit with which we face bumps in the
road.

Wherever you are, we have discovered that of all the
tools to combat depression, anxiety, negativity, and physical or emotional illness, gratitude is the most effective—
and the easiest—method. Just like mastering the craft of

writing, or learning as a student in school, we need to practice expressing gratitude for life.

Certainly, more and more these days, many of us are discovering the healing power of gratitude. It empowers us to transform challenges into opportunities. Internet social networks and blogs are abuzz with the idea of gratitude as healer. Humanity is coming to recognize the logic that it is impossible to be grateful and hateful (or angry, sad, or discouraged) at the same time.

Gratitude promotes healing, harmony, peace, and joy. It encourages forgiveness, patience, and goodwill. It is a path that opens the opportunity for us to act on the good in our lives. Science backs this up. Sonja Lyubomirsky, professor of psychology at the University of California, Riverside, says we need to make gratitude a daily practice, and it will bring healing properties to our lives.

Other experts agree.

Practicing gratitude is like exercising, says Robert Emmons, professor of psychology at the University of California, Davis. Use it, and you won't lose it, even when times are tough, as they are for many folks right now.

Both Lyubomirsky and Emmons agree: those who practice an attitude of gratitude have lower risks for many health disorders, including depression and high blood pressure.

Practicing gratitude in these systematic ways changes people by changing brains that are "wired for negativity, for noticing gaps and omissions," Emmons says. "When you express a feeling, you amplify it. When you express anger, you get angrier; when you express gratitude, you become more grateful."

GRATITUDE: THE KEY TO KICKING ADDICTION

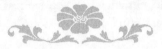

In saying "Thank you," this author found his way back to himself and to what most matters in his life.

> Gratitude is the intention to count your blessings every day, every minute, while avoiding, whenever possible, the belief that you need or deserve different circumstances.
>
> —Timothy Miller

The battle to kick an addiction is one that often creates chaos in the lives of everyone around. Even if you have never been affected by the devastation of a loved one's addiction to alcohol, illegal drugs, or prescription medication, you may know that substance abusers often replace one addiction with another. It may be food, shopping, gambling, or another drug of choice. The key to moving ahead, after battling demons and experiencing the trauma of detox, lies in ongoing support and help—and a new outlook to prevent relapse and jump-start a sober life anew.

*In this story, Alan Kaufman, author of the criti-
cally acclaimed memoir* Jew Boy *and the novel* Matches,
*reveals his descent into and recovery from alcoholism.
Kaufman, whose book* The Outlaw Bible of American
Poetry *was featured on the cover of the* New York Times
Book Review *and whose poetry was instrumental in the
development of the Spoken Word movement in literature,
shows us how he turned to the practice of gratitude to
help power his way through recovery. In finding what
he was grateful for in life, he found himself again, and is
keeping himself addiction free.*

Most mornings, Alan Kaufman admits, he doesn't bounce
out of bed happy. On the contrary, he is more likely to
wake up grumpy. As a recovering alcoholic, he knows that
many alcoholics are predisposed to negativity and self-
pity. So when Alan wakes up, he has to consciously make
an effort to lighten and brighten his mood, and push away
the heaviness. He purposefully cultivates a strategy that is
commonly recommended to those in recovery—he focuses
on what he is most grateful for in his life.

And that vital tool is giving thanks. "If we hang around
resentment, it is deadly," he explains. "Gratitude is my life
raft."

These days, even if he isn't bouncing out of bed, at least
he's grateful that he is waking up in one. When he first went
into recovery almost 20 years ago, this acclaimed novelist

and award-winning editor was living on the streets.

Raised in the Bronx, Alan had two close friends and three cousins die from heroin overdoses. And alcoholism ran in his family as well. Desperate to escape what seemed to be his destiny, he enrolled in college and focused on his dream of becoming a writer. But drinking and writing were inseparable to him—it was a badge of honor to drink, and drink heavily. Despite that, Alan managed to attend the graduate program in creative writing at Columbia University, home to a number of famous writers, and he held two executive jobs for nonprofit organizations.

He recalls those days—working hard and partying hard. Once, at a faculty party at Columbia, Alan encountered one person who wasn't drinking. "This sober person came up to me and told me that he had heard I was a very good writer," recalls Alan. "I was completely drunk, but I do remember him pointing at my glass of whiskey and saying, 'That is going to stand in your way.' "

Alan ignored the messenger. Instead, he fell into a downward spiral during this stressful period in his life. He was editing magazines, trying to raise money for foundations, and living with terrible uncertainty about his baby daughter's health.

"For the first time in my life, I was terrified," recalls Alan. "The stress of that time precipitated a spinout."

He adds: "I couldn't stop. I would vow, No more, but then find myself blacked out in doorways at four A.M. For three months, my life was like a hurricane had swept me away."

He employed many excuses in order to cope. When he passed a junkie eating out of a dumpster, he would console himself with the thought *At least I'm not doing that*. The next week, when he found himself eating someone's trash, he would think *At least I'm not lying on the street*. The following week, when he woke up in the street, he would think *At least I'm not lying in the gutter*.

His wife and child left him and moved out of the country. He lost one of his jobs, and then the other. After his unemployment checks terminated and he ran out of places to "couch-surf," he slept on the street. But his rationalizations continued. *I'm like George Orwell researching 'Down and Out in Paris and London,'* he told himself.

Then one day, Alan called a friend whom he hadn't talked to since graduate school and poured out his story. His friend put his wife on the phone, who told Alan to get in a cab and come immediately to their brownstone in Brooklyn Heights, where they were waiting on the steps. "This friend was a hugely successful screenwriter, and his wife, who was five months pregnant, was a recovering alcoholic who hadn't had a drink in five years," he remembers. "She asked me, 'Have you ever considered the possibility that you could stop drinking?' "

That one question triggered a lot of soul searching for the first time in Alan's life.

"A part of me wanted to lose everything," he recalls. "All my illusions were gone. I was no longer a high-powered executive, a parent, a writer. And when my identity was stripped to the core, I found not a great luminous truth, but only the realization that I wanted to kill myself. It was always a torment to be me, and the medicine I used to allow me to live in my skin was alcohol."

He attended his first recovery meeting and a lightbulb went on.

"People looked happy, they looked sane," he says. They were talking about drinking in ways he had never heard before. No one was pressuring him, they just told their stories. These people had been self-annihilating drinkers but they realized that they could no longer live if they continued to drink. Alcohol had been their best friend and their best friend had betrayed them.

After a week of meetings, accompanied by tremors and hallucinations, Alan became aware of the possibility of recovery. He decided to move to San Francisco. A friend lent him money that he used to buy a Greyhound bus ticket. He put his few belongings in a garbage bag and went to the station in midtown Manhattan.

AN EPIPHANY MOMENT

"As I was leaning against a pillar, I noticed an elderly woman, possibly eighty, leaning against another pillar with an identical garbage bag," he recalls. "We had both just stomped out our cigarette butts on the floor. I remember thinking that even though I'm an Ivy League graduate, there's absolutely no difference between her and me. I felt a huge surge of love and a sense of gratitude. I had been brought to the level of common humanity and it was freeing in so many ways. That was the beginning of my healing."

"After that, I continued in recovery, which gave me so many gifts, including a life that was true to who I am," says Alan. He started exploring spiritual paths and found truths that he heard in recovery. For instance, there is a Hassidic saying, "You should be grateful for everything that happens to you, even your pain." The saying suggests that you cannot think your way into right action, only act your way into right thinking. "So even if you don't feel like performing an act of service, but do it anyway, at a certain point you'll feel gratitude," explains Alan.

According to Alan, most people think you have to be grateful to begin with to perform an act of service, but it's often the other way around. "If you act in a principled way, you'll go from self-pity to a love for humanity," Alan says. "Gratitude is a direct path to love."

Gratitude saved his life and keeps on saving it, two decades later.

GRATITUDE PRACTICE
Alan meditates on a daily basis to connect to a higher

power. When he does, he asks himself, Who needs a blessing? He mentally imagines sending that person a blessing to help them through their challenges.

GRATITUDE AS A POWERFUL HEALER

*Wake at dawn with a winged heart and give thanks
for another day of loving.*

—Kahlil Gibran

*Dan Reich lives to thrive. And there is no doubt that he
has triumphed over extreme physical challenges in his
determination to move through what doctors told him
was a terminal brain tumor.*

*Throughout the last seven years, Dan has exuded a
positive determination, grace, and soulfulness that have
infused his journey through illness with hope and gratitude for every day of living. It is the power of gratefulness
for the incredible gift of life that he believes saved his.*

*Here, Dan reminds us how important it is to take care
of both our physical and emotional health and to become*

aware of what we can be grateful for. When we do, we can unlock our full healing potential.

The neurologist met Dan Reich's eyes with a neutral gaze, betraying no emotion, as she told him he had six months to live. Dan had been diagnosed with a malignant brain tumor.

"What are the chances of my making a full recovery?" Dan asked.

"I wouldn't think in terms of a full recovery," the doctor replied, and at that moment, the rest of Dan's life began.

That was almost seven years ago. Since his return to health, he describes feeling that he has been living in a state of grace, having been given the gift of a second chance at life.

"After my diagnosis, I remember feeling an unexpected calm, accepting my fate without fear, anger, or resentment," Dan says. "As I contemplated the end, I found enjoyment in things I formerly took for granted—a soak in the pool on a warm day, a walk in nearby China Camp Park—and began to feel a profound gratitude for each new day that I had the privilege to experience."

Dan had surgery to remove the tumor and numerous courses of treatment. He sought alternative therapies after his tumor returned but he continued to have daily seizures. Then he was referred to a Qigong healer located near his home in Marin County, California.

"The first time I worked with Donald Rubbo, I experienced a seizure, which he felt was a positive sign," relates Dan. "He taught me a daily meditation and movement practice, and arranged to have a monastery in Tibet chant for my well-being. On the day of the chanting, I was instructed to keep my mind free of negative thoughts, and I kept myself in a positive place for the entire day. As I fell asleep that night, I felt a pleasurable tingling sensation engulf my whole body. Five days after the chanting, I was seizure-free, and I felt my energy level increasing."

Dan was especially grateful to be able to celebrate his 25th wedding anniversary with his wife, Ellen, nine months after his diagnosis. He began to take long walks, and soon was able to return to running. A special cancer-screening blood test indicated that his body was successfully fighting off the tumor, and an MRI revealed that the tumor was shrinking. His gratitude began to shift from appreciating the time he had left to appreciating his return to health.

"After six months without a seizure, I was again able to drive, and felt a surge of gratitude for something I had always taken for granted," he says. "The next scheduled MRI confirmed that the tumor had stabilized and the seizures that accompanied it were now a thing of the past. Not only was I living on borrowed time, I was fortunate to enjoy the quality of life I had before my diagnosis, except that the enjoyment went far deeper than before. I had been given back my life with the added gifts of gratitude and perspective."

In the ensuing years, Dan has continued to experience profound gratitude for so many things he might not have had the chance to experience—recording a CD, participating in marathons for the National Brain Tumor Foundation, his children's graduations, a 30th anniversary spent in Africa—and for the smallest of things.

Dan, a musician and graphic artist, also looks for ways to express his gratitude, from performing benefit shows for Bread and Roses to meditating on Tibetan chants that seek to alleviate suffering in the world. Every breath, every moment is like a tiny gift, and he tries to honor those gifts by never forgetting how fortunate he is to be alive and realizing how precious a gift life really is.

GRATITUDE PRACTICE

In putting together the Gratitude Practices for this book, our intention is to offer simple ways you can incorporate thankfulness in your everyday lives. We believe that music is a powerful healer—it heals the heart. Olivia Newton-John, a cancer survivor who studied the work of Carolyn Myss and Dr. Deepak Chopra in her own healing, has created a CD, Grace and Gratitude, *in appreciation for the gift of life. The songs are meant for you to use as a relaxation and meditation exercise. For more information, go to* www.OliviaNewton-John.com.

LEGACY OF HOPE: DANA REEVE

The burden which is well borne becomes light.

—Ovid

One quality of most grateful people is that they don't focus so much on pain and problems. They don't dwell on their losses and are quicker to realize the blessings in even the toughest times. They tap into their families and friends during times of need, and they step back and ask themselves how they can help others in distress as well.

When Dana Reeve died of lung cancer, just before her 45th birthday, in March 2006, her family pulled together in open-ended conversations about how they could carry on her legacy of caring and compassion to give back to the world.

"My sister and Chris (Reeve) created a positive legacy," says Dr. Deborah Morosini, Dana Reeve's sister. "They showed the world that out of crisis, you can make a life; you can have a sense of humor and not fall apart. They touched so many people—people including myself who maybe looked at them and said, Okay, I can get through this, I can remain optimistic."

Certainly, Dana and Christopher Reeve had become public icons of survival, inspirations for the world to draw strength from, following the 1995 horseback riding accident that left Christopher a ventilator-dependent quadriplegic. Together, with their intensive focus on paralysis and stem cell research, the couple and the forces they rallied shone a spotlight on an injury for which research was poorly funded. They made it a cause. When Christopher died at 52, in 2004, Dana kept up the cause.

It is with that spirit of gratitude that the family moved forward to heal and to make a difference in others' lives. It is their collective belief that focusing on the positives is always beneficial, and it is especially healing during the bumpy times to be able to move toward positivity and gratitude.

In March 2009, three years almost to the date of his aunt Dana Reeve's untimely death from lung cancer, James Lichtenthal, 18, boarded a 5:30 A.M. plane to New York City from Boston, carrying expectations of hope and change to high school students and guests gathered at a rally against cancer at Fiorello LaGuardia High School of Music & Art and Performing Arts in Manhattan.

On this morning, the Weston, Massachusetts, high school senior was on a mission. Carrying T-shirts and buttons with the message to stamp out lung cancer, he arrived at the school near Lincoln Center and quickly set up his booth.

Within seconds, it was swarmed by more than 200 high school students—who quickly donned the attire and adorned themselves with the buttons: "What kills more women than breast cancer? Lung Cancer" and "Girls just want to have none: Lung Cancer."

James was at the American Cancer Society's Cancer Awareness Day to speak about the tragedy of his aunt's death, how it affected their family and indeed the world, and the lack of funding and awareness about lung cancer research and treatment today.

But most importantly, he says, he was there to show the world the positive legacy his aunt gave to him, one he says he is eternally grateful for. He wants to touch people in the way Dana and her husband, Christopher Reeve, did, showing them that when faced with crisis, you can say, Okay, I can get through this, I can remain optimistic. And that in the face of illness, you can continue to move forward with gratitude for the life you have and for the fact that there is always hope.

"I believe that it is our individual duty to make the best of what is thrown at you," says James. "Although we all live very different lives, we are all in constant search of happiness and satisfaction. If one does not come to terms with and appreciate their inner gifts, and acknowledge their character flaws, they are inhibited to find this greater goal.

"Also, if one is not grateful for what they currently have, it is difficult to build off of what they have."

Sage wisdom for a guy who goes to high school full-time, works nights as a lifeguard, and is busy exploring colleges.

"When my aunt Dana died, I decided to be proactive and do something that would help support her cause and the cause of millions throughout the world."

That is how he and his family found the way to move on.

"Acceptance of one's position in life allows us to move forward because we are doing so on a much sturdier realistic limb," says James. "Living in the now, understanding and being grateful toward and about what we currently have, and not only searching for later satisfaction but current satisfaction, is the way that I see fit to truly discover happiness and realization of one's purpose."

And so, James has become the new generation in the fight against lung cancer, with zeal and gratitude for the opportunity.

"To me it is appalling that so many people die of lung cancer," he says. "At first, all the students came up to the booth because they wanted to know if the clothes were free, and when I said yes, the clothes were gone in, like, three minutes. But then I'd ask them what they knew about lung cancer. And they were *shocked* by what I told them."

March 6th, the day after James's appearance in New York, was the third anniversary of Dana's death. She died only days before what would have been her 45th birthday, and two years after the death of her husband, "Superman," Christopher Reeve. His riding accident in 1995 resulted in his paralysis from the neck down. In the years that followed, the world watched as Dana rose to the challenge of this tragedy with the strength, grace, and compassion that everyone now knows as her hallmark.

James comes from a family of doctors. His mother is a doctor, his grandfather is a doctor. He is determined to keep speaking up about what he calls "the tremendous ignorance about the facts of lung cancer, and about its treatments. I want to help make a difference. I want to do so for my aunt, for everything she did for me. We were very close."

These days, James is exploring college opportunities. He has his sights set on the University of California at Santa Barbara. He is studying American literature, DNA/biotech investing, environmental science, and precalculus, and for his independent study he is compiling a 20-minute documentary about the trip he made with his family to President Obama's inauguration. He's also taking classical guitar and acting lessons, and going to auditions several times a week. He just finished costarring in a film his school funded about a historical museum in Weston.

"I am determined to keep trying to help people with lung cancer," he says.

GRATITUDE PRACTICE
We all know how to say "Thanks." Just saying the word to the barista at your coffeehouse, or the guy at the front desk at the gym who swipes your membership card, is a good start. It gives your gratitude muscle a workout and reminds us to thank significant others in our lives as well.

MAKING ONESELF WHOLE
THROUGH GRATITUDE

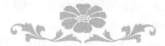

When you are grateful, fear disappears and abun-
dance appears.

—Anthony Robbins

When Angela LaPorta, of Pleasant Hill, California, does
daily chanting and a ho'oponopono *prayer, she not only*
feels grateful all the time, "life actually gets easier and I
can create what I do want with real ease," she says.

But it's when she's on a roll of abundance, peace, and
happiness that she sometimes forgets to practice gratitude.

"Most of the time I will start up again at the first sign
of trouble, but sometimes I don't," Angela says. "It's at
those times that I can't believe the amount of crap that
shows up in my life. And then it's really hard to get back to
daily chanting and repeating the ho'oponopono *prayer."*

In late summer of 2008, Angela LaPorta's life was better than it had been in years. In spite of a debilitating menopause, she was finding help in homeopathy treatments.

"My business was finally where I wanted it to be and my nine-year love relationship was still going strong," she recalls. "I felt so optimistic and abundant and powerful."

In September 2008, she was married and launched into the massive project of decorating her house. Her business as a massage therapist and aesthetician was booming and she had a waiting list of clients.

But all the busyness started taking its toll, and Angela found herself constantly fatigued. The first thing to go: she gave up her daily practices of gratitude. Because she was so busy, she hadn't even noticed she was forgetting.

Then the busyness of the holidays descended, and she spiraled into stress overload.

"With aging in-laws and a sibling who's always in some kind of trouble, I had more challenges than I could handle, especially without the help of my chanting and prayer," Angela admits. "By the end of January, I was falling apart."

A series of alarming events occurred: Her business dropped off. The business owner she shared space with got involved in an illegal situation. She had computer trouble. And she had a major setback in her homeopathic treatment.

"My computer printer died and my computer was so old that I needed to buy a new one just to accommodate an upgraded printer. I bought a used computer on eBay and it wound up needing to be repaired. The computer still had repair insurance on it, but it lapsed the day that I called in the problem.

"I was at the point in my homeopathic treatment where I took a potent formula that was to reverse many, if not all, of my symptoms. Although I was told that initially the formula might increase my symptoms, I was not prepared for the two weeks that followed. Depression and rage mixed in with sleeplessness and high anxiety, and hot flashes that left me soaking wet ensued.

"I became immersed in this dark place. I just wanted to curl up and hide."

Angela spent almost two months feeling off-kilter. Thankfully, and gradually, her problems began to resolve.

"But I was so tense from the situation at my office that I couldn't relax," she says. "Finally, I was able to talk myself back into chanting and prayer."

And that is when she was reminded of the tremendous power of gratitude in her life. Gratitude became nothing short of a miraculous cure.

"All it took was one hour and I felt so much calmer," she confides. "My body relaxed and the stress in my mind just melted away." Even though she is still dealing with the legal ramifications of her business shared-space neighbor, gratitude calmed the frenzy.

"As always, when I come back to this place, I wonder how it is that I stopped doing what makes me so grateful for the wonderful life I have," she reflects. "Although I use two different spiritual practices, when I use them together they are the most powerful personal means of transformation I have ever experienced."

GRATITUDE PRACTICE
Angela practices the Nichiren Buddhist chant "Nam myoho renge kyo." (For information on how to do this chant, go to www.sgi-usa.org.) *Information on the ancient Hawaiian practice of* ho'oponopono *can be found in the book* Zero Limits, *by Joe Vitale.*

TEN WAYS TO GET MORE ENERGY
BY BEING THANKFUL

Anne Naylor, a personal motivation coach, author, and Huffington Post blogger, advises that we all carry a precious resource with us: thankfulness. No one can take it away. However, you can either enhance or diminish your awareness of it. Here, Anne offers 10 tips for becoming grateful—and energized in that process.

1. **Gratitude journal**

   Keep a gratitude journal. At the end of each day, write five things you feel grateful for from the day: a smile from a stranger, a hug from your child, an unexpected compliment, a good meal, a moment of laughter with a friend.

2. **Before sleeping**

   Go to bed with a smile, thinking about all you appreciate in your life. Breathe deeply and relax as you do so.

3. **Gratitude dance**

   Take a few minutes and begin your day with a gratitude dance. Start your day as you would intend it to be. If your energy is flagging during the day—do it again. It will probably make you laugh, and that will energize and refresh you.

4. **Appreciate family, friends and co-workers**
    Bring to mind those close to you whom you love, and
    how thankful you are that they are part of your life.
    Make a note in your journal of your special people
    and why you appreciate them.

5. **Express appreciation**
    At home, work, or in your community, take a little
    time to communicate your appreciation to those you
    value—in person, over the phone, by e-mail.

    > *In everyone's life, at some time, our inner
    > fire goes out. It is then burst into flame by
    > an encounter with another human being.
    > We should all be thankful for those people
    > who rekindle the inner spirit.*
    >
    > —*Albert Schweitzer*

6. **Midday break**
    Take a short walk and count your blessings, feeling
    grateful as you do so. You will come back inspired and
    enthusiastic for the afternoon.

7. **Blessings in disguise**
    When you are going through a tough time, it is harder
    to feel grateful. However, when you do, the results can
    be amazing. When things are not going your way, or
    the way you had intended, declare them a "blessing in

disguise" and be grateful for them. This simple shift in attitude will make you a winner, no matter what happens.

8. **Gratitude gathering**
Bring a group of friends together for a gratitude gathering and recount the things you are grateful for. Conclude with a celebratory potluck meal.

9. **Nature walk**
Take a walk in nature and notice the beauty around you. Beauty might be in something very simple like a leaf, a bird in flight, sunlight on dew, an elegant branch of a tree, the color of the sky, the crunch of gravel, or the softness of grass beneath your feet. Allow yourself to feel the beauty and your gratitude for it.

10. **Be grateful for you**
Last but absolutely not least, take a moment to notice the goodness of your intent; the caring you express to others; the endeavors you take to be true to your ideals, even at difficult times. Be grateful for and bless your qualities and strengths. There is no one else quite like you. Honor and appreciate yourself.

To read more of Anne Naylor's writing, check out her blog at http://www.huffingtonpost.com/anne-naylor/

CHAPTER TWO
GRATEFUL FOR THE GOOD LIFE: KEYS TO LIVING YOUR LIFE WITH GRATITUDE

The winds of grace blow all the time. All we need to do is set our sails.

—Sri Ramakrishna Paramahamsa

There is an expression that says if you want to turn your life around, try thankfulness. Finding reasons to be grateful every day is the key to living an abundant life.

We all have experienced being around people who find beauty at every turn of the road. They are really and truly grateful for each and every encounter—the smile on a stranger's face, the kindness of the barista. When we are with these people, it sets our vibrations higher; it makes us aware that we are responsible for attracting all those things that will make our lives more complete.

Through the stories in this chapter, we've found people

who have inspired us with their attitudes of gratitude. We share their secrets, to encourage you, the reader, to tap into your own inner fount of thankfulness and to be more conscious of all the gifts in your life.

We've made some observations on the qualities of a grateful person, and invite you to undertake the spirit of thankfulness and experience the empowerment that follows.

Grateful people, we've discovered, seem to be more resilient. They seem to have an easier time overcoming obstacles. Grateful people are more appreciative of others, and in being so, more willing to be of service to give back in gratitude. They realize how others have helped them and they don't take anything for granted.

Many look at grateful people and say they are lucky or blessed, or just fortunate. Rather, such people understand that gratitude is a signature strength. They make a point to train their gratitude muscle every day, just as if it were their heart, or their mind, or their body on a treadmill.

The result: grateful people have a sense of wonder and look at the world through the eyes of astonishment and joy. By focusing on what they have, and being grateful for it, they bypass feelings of neediness, anger, or greediness.

Grateful people express their gratitude by being thankful. Gratitude resides in their hearts and souls. In turn, grateful people often express their thankfulness through their own actions and deeds.

Here, meet some wonderful gratitude guides who live the way Meister Eckhart suggested: "If the only prayer you said in your whole life was 'Thank you,' that would suffice."

GLORY BE: GIVING THANKS FOR SODA, TOOTSIE ROLLS, AND WHAT LIES AHEAD

Expressing gratitude is a natural state of being and reminds us that we are all connected.

—*Valerie Elster*

It's no secret that practicing gratitude as a daily ritual rewires your brain to see the cup half full. You'll be happier, healthier, and more grateful for the blessings in your life.

Have you ever noticed the way it feels to be around grateful people? You feel energized, alive, and inspired to give thanks yourself for the friends, families, and community members that make a difference in your daily living. When we're grateful, we reach out to help others in need, instead of focusing on our own woes, anger, or resentments. Here, we see how we all need a little "George

Bailey" epiphany moment to wake us up when we are immersed in our daily living. Anthony Migyanka teaches us to "Give thanks, be happy."

Call Anthony Migyanka a modern-day Jimmy Stewart (George Bailey in *It's a Wonderful Life*), because he has figured out what his life would be like without the people and things he may have taken for granted. Coincidentally growing up just 30 miles from the famous star's hometown, in western Pennsylvania, Migyanka has made it a daily practice to keep a list of what he is thankful for in his life—and for things that he hopes to happen. His practice seems to be working.

These days, the Irving, Texas, investor relations specialist is reveling in the fruits of that attention to gratitude and the success he believes it has brought to his personal and professional life. He has appeared as an expert on "Cavuto on Business" and he has also given expert commentary on several national TV shows and in the *Washington Post*.

"I have used spoken gratitude in my daily life to produce much success and contentment," Anthony says. "First of all, in my business, after I decide on a course of action, I say thank you for the results not yet obtained, for the future gratitude of today."

He laughs when he explains that he speaks clearly but "usually with no one around," rattling off his list of to-be-thankful-for future events. The checklist may include Thank you for a productive meeting, Thank you for letting my company find the right vendor, or Thank you for a job well done.

Giving thanks in his personal life is an especially profound daily practice for Anthony.

Every evening, when he is tucking into bed his two children, ages three and six, they share their prayers together. "We say a 'Glory Be,' an 'Our Father,' and then we say our 'Thank you' prayers separately. We each take a minute to say what we were thankful for that day, in our own words. My son usually says thank you for a soda, if he got one that day, or a Tootsie Roll, or thank you for letting us go to the zoo. My daughter usually says thank you for this nice house or my dolly, or something like that. Only after we say thank you do we add a special intention (occasionally), for something to come to pass in the future, and we give thanks that it will."

Counting his blessings every day gives Anthony the energy to handle all the challenges that lie ahead.

"Using spoken gratitude frequently, daily, has really made a difference in my life," he says. "It has made me calmer, less fearful, and happier. After the spoken gratitude, it's like I can move on to the business at hand, and be present, as the saying goes, and not work with a divided mind on things."

GRATITUDE PRACTICE

Write a letter of gratitude to the people in your everyday life who make a difference—the mailman, a grocery clerk, or the greeter at your gym. Tell your friends about their places of business or their great service so their businesses can grow.

SECRET SHOPPER: SAYING THANKS TO THOSE
WHO HAVE ANSWERED THE CALL TO DUTY

*Gratefulness—the simple response of our heart to
this life in all its fullness—goes beyond boundaries
of creed, age, vocation, gender, and nation.*

—J. Robert Moskin

When we realize that life flows through our attitudes and
actions, we create a channel for the universe to move
through us to connect with others. Our growth is growth
for everyone.

Here, we see how the compassion of Kelleigh Nelson
radiates and multiplies in abundance and opportunities for others. Kelleigh reaches out to help the soldiers
who are risking their lives for our freedom. Through her
thankfulness for these soldiers' service to others, for their
strength and courage, Kelleigh shows them that someone
cares.

Before maneuvering her cart through the Fresh Market grocery store checkout line, Kelleigh Nelson makes sure the sandwiches and drinks of the guy or young woman in the desert camouflage and tan boots are paid for. It's a quick heads-up signal the clerk's have come to know, as they bag the groceries and announce to the surprised military person: "A grateful American has already paid for this."

This twice-a-week lunchtime gesture in Knoxville, Tennessee, is Kelleigh's way of saying "Thank you" for the service of soldiers and other military personnel who have risked their lives to defend ours.

"They usually never know who paid for their bill," she enthuses. "But I watch from a distance and I've seen the smiles, the looks on their faces, the gratitude they show and the thanks they give to the clerk to send on to the anonymous bill payer—me. It's actually thrilling and I know it lifts their spirits when they go back to the troops and tell them what happened. It's a little thing, and I've never paid more than fourteen dollars, but it's so worth it to tell them 'Thank you' for their commitment, their service, and their sacrifices."

Extending gratitude to the military has been a life-time tradition for Nelson's family. The 62-year-old grandmother of three remembers when she was a little girl and her maternal grandfather, who served in the Army in World

War I, always urged the family to find ways to ensure that the troops were thanked. Ditto for her paternal grandfather, who served in the Army Cavalry in both world wars, retiring as a colonel. Her uncles, also in the military, carried on the practice of gratitude, and when Kelleigh married her husband, Larry, it became part of their new family's mission.

Sending e-mails to Larry's Uncle Gale, who was in the Special Forces in Vietnam and at Ft. Bragg, they would get a list of soldiers who needed help the most and send checks so Gale could buy the soldiers phone cards to call home.

THE RIPPLE EFFECT: A CIRCLE OF THANKS

When the uncle died in February 2008, the Nelsons received a folded flag that had been flown over Baghdad and a certificate of appreciation for the donations.

"To say we wept at their wonderful note and gift of thanks is an understatement," says Nelson. "Even today it brings tears to my eyes. We've never flown that flag because those men folded it for us. We cherish it."

Though she prefers to be an anonymous benefactor in her secret shopping adventures, her cover has been broken by observant servicemen.

"One day I was in line and saw a soldier in another line, so I told the bag man to quickly run over and tell the clerk that I'd pay for the soldier's purchases," she says. "Unfortunately, he said it to the clerk out loud, telling her and the soldier that I was paying for the purchase. The soldier smiled and thanked me, and I was so embarrassed that he knew that I hurried outside to my car. He came running outside behind me and was screaming, 'Thank you so much and God bless you' and waving. But I really don't like being 'caught.' "

SIGN OF THE TIMES: A SIMPLE WAY TO SAY THANK YOU TO OUR TROOPS

When Scott Truit was traveling around the country, he began approaching soldiers in airports, thanking them for serving America. Several times, he recalls, the servicemen and women appeared slightly uncomfortable, even though he knows they appreciated it, and he felt good extending his gratitude.

Thinking it would be nice if civilians had a gesture or sign they could use to say "Thank you" to soldiers, he created one. He founded The Gratitude Campaign to spread the sign of "Thank you."

The sign is intended to communicate "Thank you from the bottom of my heart."

To make the sign, simply place your hand on your heart as though you're saying the Pledge of Allegiance. Then pull your hand down and out, bending at the elbow (not the wrist), stopping for a moment at about the belly button with your hand flat, palm up, angled toward the person you're thanking.

thank you.

The sign is actually borrowed from sign language used to communicate "Thank you" for the deaf. According to Norman Heimgartner, Ed.D., author of *Behavioral Traits of Deaf Children* and former professor of education at the University of Puget Sound, this sign originated in France in the late 1700s and was published in *Théorie des Signes*, a dictionary of signs by the Abbé Sicard. The sign was brought to the United States in 1816 by the Reverend Thomas Hopkins Gallaudet, founder of American School for the Deaf, who later modified it to start at the chin rather than at the heart. That sign is now the standard sign for "Thank you" in American Sign Language. The original sign, starting at the heart, is less commonly known today and might now be considered "slang."

Check out the powerful video on The Gratitude Campaign's website: www.gratitudecampaign.org.

BLESSED TO BE HERE RIGHT NOW: BEING GRATEFUL FOR THE SMALLEST THINGS

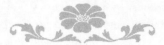

Let us be grateful to people who make us happy—
they are the charming gardeners who make our
souls blossom.

—Marcel Proust

Dena Dyer has an incredible appreciation for life. She
believes that all human beings are connected and she is
determined to pass on to her own children a legacy of
grace and gratitude she received from her mother.

That's her intention. Recently she was delighted when
her young son asked her to guide him to express his
own gratitude for "Santa, Baby Jesus, and Mommy and
Daddy." Her story shows how an attitude of gratitude is
one of the important lessons and legacies we as parents
can pass on to the next generation—if we are bound by
gratitude and grace to speak of it and incorporate it into
our connections with others.

* * *

Dena Dyer's five-and-a-half-year-old son Jordan saw his mom reading the book *Ferris Wheels, Daffodils and Hot Fudge Sundaes*, by Laura Jensen Walker. This gratitude journal, which was inspired by Walker's bout with breast cancer, consists of blank pages to write on, quotes and scriptures about thankfulness, and her own lists of things—both big and little—she's grateful for.

The little boy asked if he could write in it, and here's what he recorded (spelling errors and translations included): "I'm thankful for ... Santa, baby Jesus, mommy and dade, mi (my) house, or (our) bones, mi presents, or hort (our heart), luv fum (from) momy and dady, for God, apol jows (apple juice), and I am gad dit we r nt mosdrs (I am glad that we are not monsters)."

Jordan's creative list inspired Dena to write down some of the things she's thankful for, most notably her mom, who made her write thank-you notes after every holiday—before she played with her gifts—and who wrote affirming letters listing the things about her daughter she was thankful for.

"Come to think of it, my mother was an excellent model of thanksgiving," says Dena. "Even as she was going through a lengthy illness, she kept a great attitude. And Jordan's desire to create his own journal page reminded me that gratitude—like many of the attributes we want (or don't want!) our children to develop, can be taught by example."

"This, surely, is the most valuable legacy we can pass on to the next generation," writes Arthur Gordon in *A Touch of Wonder*. "Not money, houses or heirlooms, but a capacity for wonder and gratitude, a sense of aliveness and joy. Why don't we work harder at it? Probably because, as Thoreau said, "Our lives are frittered away by detail." There are times when we don't have the awareness or the selflessness or the energy." Dena is determined to continue cultivating her own attitude of gratitude so she can continue to sow seeds of gratitude in her children.

GRATITUDE PRACTICE

We teach our children good manners and conventional gratitude: to say "Thank you" when they receive a present. We may even teach them gratitude out of guilt: "We've sacrificed so much for you, and you don't even appreciate it!" This imparts a sense of duty and obligation. Instead, ask your children to make a list of what they're grateful for, or begin each meal with a recitation of things to be thankful for. This will help them on their path to a more fulfilled life.

REAL, SIMPLE GRATITUDE

Patti Haare, mom of two from Palatine, Illinois, says: "I am thankful (and I am totally serious about this) that Morningstar Farms makes veggie sausage with maple flavoring. They always had great veggie sausage, but the maple makes them so yummy. It's a small thing, but when you're a vegetarian and love the taste and smell of sausage—it's monumental!"

FINDING THANKS AT TARGET

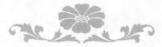

When we recognize the Divine Presence every-where, then we know that it responds to us and that there is a Law of God, a Law of Love, forever giving of itself to us.

—Ernest Holmes

Giving thanks is an important part of all faiths, and an important lesson all parents want to teach their children. But it can sometimes be hard for parents to know how to guide their children in prayers of thanksgiving.

When we open our hearts to divine guidance, often the teacher or teaching moment comes to us. We just need to surrender our own need to orchestrate these moments, and pay attention to the circumstances around us.

Here, during an ordinary shopping excursion for cleaning products, Camerone Thorson discovers that her young son Nicholas has found his own unique way to spot the things he is grateful for in his life, and to give voice through his own concerns, hopes, and gratitude.

Camerone Thorson and her 10-year-old son Nicholas were at Target surrounded by the frenzy of holiday shoppers and the sights and smells of Christmas—life-size snowmen, glittery snowflakes, and red-and-green-striped cardboard stockings dangling from the ceiling. It was the beginning of the holiday shopping season and the aisles were a virtual Toyland, chock full with merchandise designed to entice the young and old alike: books, balls, toys, bicycles, scooters, MP3 players in every size and shape imaginable. Everywhere the mom and son duo turned, they were reminded: only 24 shopping days 'til Christmas.

With her son at her side pointing out "suggested" gift ideas for Mom/Santa to put under the tree, Camerone remembers Nicholas thinking of others too: "Hey, Mom, Trevor would love the new NFL '09 game for the Nintendo Wii."

"Mmm, I nodded absently, trying to make sure I focused on my list at hand," Camerone remembers. Nicholas again piped in: "I bet Dad would love that World of Warcraft extension pack."

"I'm sure he would, dear," she remembers answering, trying to steer the cart away from the video games and closer to the cleaning supplies, which were the real reason they were in the store in the first place.

Nicholas gave her a knowing smile. She gave him a one-handed hug and continued to beeline the cart away from the pricey video games.

As they made their way through the throngs of mothers anxiously trying to peel little hands away from all the enticing objects calling to them, Camerone and Nicholas noticed a young girl with a swollen face and hands sitting in an electric wheelchair. She had a pink-and-white-striped cap on her head and a tube snaking across her lap.

Camerone says the girl looked about 10 or 11 and had blue eyes sunk deep into her pale face. Walking alongside the wheelchair and talking to the girl was an older woman with gray hair and what Camerone describes as "a haunted look."

"She—the older woman—was talking to the little girl in a sweet, lyrical voice about various gift ideas for the holidays," says Camerone. "The young girl's feet peeked out from beneath a candy-cane-red blanket. They were covered in green socks with little bows on them. Somehow the pert little bows seemed out of place with the rest of the scene, which in some ways, at least to me, felt surreal."

Nicholas and Camerone made their way to the aisle with bleach and sponges. When they were safely out of earshot, Nicholas asked, "Mom, did you see that girl in the wheelchair?"

"I did," she replied.

"What do you think is wrong with her?" Nicholas asked.

"Well," Camerone said, "I'm not sure, honey. I can guess that she has a knit cap on her head because she has undergone some kind of chemotherapy or radiation and her hair may have fallen out."

Nicholas grabbed his mom's arm. "Is she going to die?"

"I don't know, dear. Hopefully she will be cured, but who knows?"

By now they had navigated past the rows of house-cleaning supplies and were rolling by the toy section. The shelves were bulging with Legos, baby dolls, wooden blocks, Nerf guns—the supply and the shelves seemed endless.

Camerone remembers thinking *Things and more things.*

She recounts, "But the little girl's face was haunting me, making all this madness to acquire more things seem rather pointless in the bigger scheme of life."

Nicholas said in a soft voice, "That must be really sad for her mom."

"What do you mean?" Camerone asked.

"Well, I'm sure it feels really bad for the little girl. I mean, she looked about my age, Mom. But imagine how a parent would feel watching their child suffer and be so sick. I think it is harder for the parent," Nicholas explained.

"I looked at my son, tousled the top of his toffee-colored

hair, and gently kissed him on the cheek," Camerone says. "I told him, 'You are an amazing little boy, Nicholas.' Now it was my voice crackling like static."

He looked up at her and gave her a smile. His eyes were as moist as hers.

They finished their browsing and made their way to the exit. On their way out they saw the girl in the wheelchair once more. She had several toys in her lap and a smile on her face.

"My son and I looked at each other and instinctively reached for each other's hand as we walked out into the early morning sunshine," says Camerone.

GRATITUDE PRACTICE

Sit down with your child and ask him or her to create a prayer of thankfulness. Provide a simple starting point: "Thank you for..." Then ask your child to draw a picture to go with the prayer.

KEEP ON PUSHING ON: RECOGNIZING THE SUPPORT WE RECEIVE FROM OTHERS

Happiness cannot be traveled to, owned, earned, worn or consumed. Happiness is a spiritual experience of living every minute with love, grace and gratitude.

—Denis Waitley

Ann Mehl learned early on to see the reasons to be thankful in the simplest yet perhaps most significant moments in her life—the moments where family members, friends, and, later, strangers and others stepped forward to give her a gentle push to follow her dreams and achieve a life that was all it could be for her.

Now she spends her days reaching back to do the same for others. To feel gratitude is a gift; to enact it is generous and a way to express our thankfulness; and to live gratitude is to touch a higher being and all that is life-giving in the universe.

On a run through Central Park in New York, Ann Mehl noticed a young father helping his son as they both rode bicycles. She couldn't help but smile as she watched the dad push his boy along, ever so gently coaxing him up the hill. It was a steep incline, so the little guy needed multiple shoves to reach the top, where he was then able to pedal over the crest and down the other side.

The sight brought Ann back to her own childhood. When she was four years old, her father took her to the nearby ski resort. As she was too small to ride the chair lift, her dad tied a rope around his waist and single-handedly pulled her up the bunny slope—"My very own ski lift," she remembers.

Once she reached the top of the hill, she'd turn around; he'd untie the knot and give a little prod to the skis to get them moving for the ride down. Then he'd walk patiently back down the hill, where the dad and daughter duo would repeat the exercise again and again.

When Ann was learning to ride a two-wheeler for the first time, she can remember her older brother Michael holding on to the seat until she was confident enough to ride solo. When she was ready, he nudged her forward and let go while she biked on her own for the first time.

"There is a photo of that exact moment, and if you look closely you can see his guiding hand launching me, sans training wheels, into the great blue yonder," she remembers.

She adds, "Many times in my life, I have received the 'loving push' from others who cared for me: my mom, leading me into kindergarten with her hand on my shoulder; my sister Maureen, proudly walking behind me on a tour of her office as she introduced me to co-workers on visitors' day; my brother John, showing me how to swim underwater in the backyard pool; Walter, my second-eldest sibling, encouraging me as I considered the option to attend a college out of state."

There was always lots of support, she says, "and that was just from my immediate family." There were also teachers, friends, and other mentors along the way—all of them ready with a helping hand when Ann needed it.

That, in a way, is what she tries to do in her coaching practice today, she says. "Though the setting may be more formalized, the goal is always the same—a loving push to aid others in discovering and affirming their own inner abilities." She adds, "I am lucky. I feel grateful to have been given a leg up so often over the years that it is a privilege to pass it on whenever the opportunity arises.

"I don't know if that boy in Central Park will remember every detail of the afternoon when I watched his father push him up the hill. Perhaps he wasn't even aware of the push that got him there. Most of us are not. But we'd miss it if it wasn't there."

GRATITUDE PRACTICE

Pay it forward. Select someone who needs a gesture of kindness or something kind that someone once gave to you. With gratitude for what was given to you, reach out and give back. It can be a simple gesture, like sending a card. Or calling someone who is sick and saying you care. Or teaching a child to ride a bike.

CHAPTER THREE
GRATITUDE AS A SPIRITUAL PRACTICE

*We all have angels guiding us. They look after us.
They heal us, touch us, and comfort us with invisible warm hands. What will bring their help? Asking. Giving thanks.*

—Sophy Burnham

In all our lives, we experience mysterious happenings. Some call them coincidence. Others, synchronicity. And others, God.

But when you look at the world through the lens of gratefulness and thanks for what is, life becomes an answered prayer. Grace steps in and we develop a faith that hope is possible.

Grace and gratitude can be spiritual forces that propel us ahead. They guide us, and we can learn to call on the energy of this life force. We realize we are never alone. We can move out of our own way, and we make room for the blessings in our life to flow.

In the stories in this chapter, we explore how gratitude can be used as a powerful spiritual tool in our lives. We learn to begin our days praying for the gift of gratitude to see the blessings in our lives. Then we need to go about our lives being receptive and alert to the movement of grace and gratitude in them. The more we do this, the more a kind of magnetic force moves into place to draw blessings into our lives.

WE ARE OUR STORIES: THE GIFT OF LISTENING

The most powerful moral influence is example.
                                                    —Huston Smith

Knowing how to spot the moments when we are moved to grow spiritually and emotionally is important to living life with a spirit of gift and gratitude. And recognizing the deeper meanings when a teacher shares what he has learned can open the way to profound insight and significance.

Here, author Phil Cousineau, author of The Way Things Are: Conversations with Huston Smith on The Spiritual Life, *shares what he continues to learn from Huston Smith, the preeminent scholar of world religions. Smith's documentary films on Hinduism, Sufism, and*

Tibetan Buddhism have all won awards, and in 1996 he was featured on Bill Moyers's five-part PBS special The Wisdom of Faith with Huston Smith." *He has taught religion and philosophy at MIT, Syracuse University, and the University of California at Berkeley.*

Phil Cousineau, host of Global Spirit TV and bestselling author of more than 20 books, an award-winning documentary filmmaker and screenwriter, popular lecturer, travel leader, and storyteller, says one of the most gratifying moments he has ever experienced with Huston Smith over the years they have been friends and colleagues took place on the last evening of the December 1999 World Parliament of Religions in Cape Town, South Africa.

"We had traveled there with eight Native American spiritual leaders, as part of a delegation and film team, to allow them to share the story of the troubled state of religious freedom for native peoples," says Phil.

That evening had been cleared so that all of the participants could attend the signature speech by the former freedom fighter and President of South Africa, Nelson Mandela.

"Dame Fortune smiled on us, and we were able to sit only a few rows from the stage, but in deference to Huston's hearing problem I tried repeating the opening words of Mandela's speech in his ear," Phil says. "After a few failed attempts to pick up my whispers, Huston raised his hand, signaling me to stop, and whispered back, "It is enough for me to be within Mr. Mandela's *darshan*."

Phil watched Huston out of the corner of his eye for the rest of the speech, in which Mandela credited his spiritual upbringing as the source of his indomitable courage in withstanding his 27 years of imprisonment by the apartheid government.

"What struck me was the utter raptness of Huston's attention, the dignity of his bearing as he practiced the ancient Indian ritual of *darshan*, which means sitting quietly and humbly in the presence of someone whom you revere, growing simply from being there," says Phil.

He adds: "Thinking back on that evening, I recall rereading the splendid opening chapter of his seminal book, *The World's Religions*, as part of my preparation for the week's filming in Cape Town. Late one night in our hotel, I underlined the following passage, in which Smith likens the voices of the religions to a choir and asks, 'Does one faith carry the lead, or do the parts share in counterpoint and antiphony where not in full-throated chorus?' We cannot know. All we can do is try to listen carefully and with full attention to each voice in turn as it addresses the divine."

For that day, Phil is forever grateful.

"The gift not only of inspired oratory but also of listening well—these are the traits of the truly wise soul," says Phil. "I watched Huston enact both when we filmed him interviewing Native American spiritual leader, author, and political activist Winona LaDuke in Cape Town. In response to LaDuke's impassioned remarks about the continuing relevance of the old ways of her ancestors, Huston affirmed her point of view, then contrasted it with his own experience: 'I am too often criticized for calling for a return to a nonexistent golden age,' he said, 'but that's totally wrong. I am interested in what was true in the past, what is true now, and what will be true in the future. In short, I am interested in what is timeless.' "

Finally, perhaps the simplest and yet most characteristic moment of gratitude with Huston took place one morning when Phil was to interview him at his home in Berkeley, California, in May 2002.

"Knowing that we had planned to address the timely but combustible issue of how much—more or less—religion matters after the tragic events of September 11, 2001, Huston excused himself for a few minutes so that he could sit on the sundeck of his house," Phil recalls. "He needed to 'put his mind around it,' as he is fond of describing his meditations on important issues. When he returned to the living room to commence the interview, he sat down in his favorite chair, and as my producer and cameraman, Gary Rhine, assembled the equipment, Huston turned to my six-year-old son, Jack, who had accompanied us for the morning. Jack was sitting quietly on the nearby couch, drawing in his notebook, and it seemed to me then that something about his quiet concentration amid the chaos of a film shoot touched Huston's heart.

"With an impish smile, as if he were going to spring a surprise on him, Huston leaned over, and recalling one of Jack's middle names, addressed him as 'Blue.' Then he asked in his inimitable sing-song manner, 'Jack Blue, do you know the song Old Dog Blue?' Jack nodded sweetly at the play on words. 'Good!' Huston said, happily, and then began to sing that song in a raspy but tender voice."

Phil remembers that "as Huston sang his eyes locked on Jack's, as if there were no one else in the room. My son's shoulders rose and fell, like they do when he is almost giddy with happiness. By the time Huston came to the last few words of the song, Jack was in a rapture. But I am convinced his mood wasn't merely due to the extra attention he was getting. His response came from a flash of boyish pride that Huston had recalled his rather colorful middle name and that he had made a playful connection with an old (what else?) blues song just to please him."

Phil adds: "Perhaps Huston only wished for him to feel as much at home as the adults in the room, and only had reached back into the archives of his ample memory to recall a little ditty with the world blue in it. But then and there it occurred to me that I had just witnessed a sterling example of why Huston Smith has become one of the most beloved teachers of our time. One of his sagely secrets is that he treats everyone alike—children and adults, struggling students and esteemed leaders—with respect for their being singular souls. It is his way to greet everyone he encounters on the road of life, in the hallowed tradition of the Old Testament and ancient Greek myths, as if they might be angels or gods in disguise.

"As the song came to an end, and Huston smiled a smile as wide as the Jordan River, I recalled his beaming face at the end of one of his lectures at UCLA. Triumphantly, he repeated something he had recently heard from a rabbi, that it is an ancient belief that each of us has an angel marching in front of us in life, shouting exultantly, 'Make way, make way for the image of God!'

"These moments have taught me that the way things are for Huston Smith is sacred not only under exalted circumstances, such as in an ashram in India or an international conference of religion scholars in Cape Town, but in everyday life with everyday people."

And they teach us not to be ungrateful for the way things *aren't*, not to wait until things are perfect, not to wait for paradise on earth, but to be grateful in the here and now for those fleeting moments of joy, happiness, and beauty.

THE POWER OF PRAYER AND GRATITUDE

A merry heart does good like a medicine.

—*Proverbs 17:22*

Gratitude, which we define as a felt sense of wonder, thankfulness, and appreciation for life, is not something to just be practiced in good times. Just ask Sylvia Bambola of Bradenton, Florida. When her daughter became seriously ill during her second pregnancy, Sylvia and her family realized that like her daughter Gina's weakened immune system, they needed to strengthen their spirits and call on a higher power to combat the disease of hopelessness and fear brought on by the physical illness.

They refused to be gratitude-deprived and to let the threat of illness cause them to suffer and lose their faith *that all will be well; they resolved to give thanks for the power of God they believed was working in their lives through the adversity.*

Fifty years ago, Abraham Maslow, the father of humanistic psychology, also recognized the power of gratitude to recharge the soul: he described the capacity to "appreciate again and again, freshly and naively, the basic goods of life with awe, pleasure, wonder, and even ecstasy, however stale these experiences may have become to others" as a central gift for people he called "self-actualizers," people who believe in the power of the spirit to heal body and soul.

Is there power in an attitude of gratitude? The kind of power that can change things? Sylvia Bambola is sure of it. A few years ago her daughter Gina, then seven months pregnant, ended up with ulcerative colitis. A "bad clam" started the downward spiral. A mistake in medication fueled the illness.

"Oh, how sick she was!" remembers Sylvia. "Skin and bones and weak as a kitten. She lost weight, became anemic and too weak and tired to care for her toddler and new baby. Gina tried different alternative treatments. But for every step forward, she took three backward."

Then came the shift. Gina copied Scriptures on 3x5 cards and tacked them to the wall in her bathroom, reminding her to keep focused on God, and "in everything, give thanks."

"The family began to give thanks for the small victories: no additional weight loss that week, a slight cessation in the pain in her side," Sylvia says. "We were learning to employ gratitude to help her heal."

And so it went, week after week, month after month, for three years. "We were praising God for each and every victory, no matter how small, and asking for His grace in the defeats," she says. "Yes, the setbacks were bitterly painful. But setbacks are easier to face when clothed in gratitude. We began to view these setbacks as pieces of a puzzle, and we assured each other that with each piece we were closer to finding a solution."

Most victories are hard fought, and Gina's were no different. Inch by inch, she battled her way back to health.

Today, though she is still on medication, Gina is healthy. She leads an active life caring for her husband, children, and home, volunteering at church and school. Sylvia knows God's hand was in it but wonders whether Gina would have been so open to God's healing touch if her gratitude was lacking. Or if she had not been grateful for each blessing God bestowed.

"Gratitude keeps hope alive," she says. "It creates joy in the heart."

GRATITUDE PRACTICE

Pray for someone else. During difficult times when a loved one, a friend, or even a stranger you know is suffering from illness or loss, make it a practice to pray for them. Find a quiet place to sit down and write a prayer for the other person. Composing the words of the prayer helps align that person with a higher power. Then give thanks for your own health and blessings.

GRATITUDE AS PAUSE, AND PRAYER

Renee Tilton borrows a daily gratitude practice she witnessed her father, Richard Tilton, of Arizona, practicing.

"I noticed that each morning after he went outside to get the newspaper, he stood for a few minutes quietly looking up at the sky and reflecting," Renee says. "When I asked him what he was thinking, he said that he starts his mornings by appreciating God's beautiful creation and thinking, *This is the day the Lord has made. Let us rejoice and be glad in it.*"

Renee adds, "As I lock the front door as I'm leaving my house, I pause for a moment to thank God for my home and family, then I look up at the beautiful sky and thank Him for a wonderful day. It puts me in the right frame of mind to start each day."

SEEKING THE SACRED IN THE ORDINARY

Whoever you are—I have always depended on the kindness of strangers.

—Blanche DuBois (in A Streetcar Named Desire, *by Tennessee Williams)*

MARY BETH'S STORY

It happened on the commuter train. I was in the middle of a very difficult time. I had never felt so alone and afraid in my life. I rested my head against the window, wiping away the tears and hoping no one saw me.

Suddenly, someone tapped me on the shoulder and handed me a hand-drawn note.

Scrawled in pen were a rainbow and a sun and the words: "I see you there crying. Know that the sun will come out again, and that you are never alone. You do not know me, but I will pray for you."

I only saw the well-manicured hand of a woman. But I never even saw the women's face. She disappeared almost instantly. But I knew, in that moment, that no matter what happened to me or my children again, we would never be alone. I had witnessed firsthand the power of one person's prayer for another at work—big time.

I had seen the power of the kindness of strangers in our lives. And I believed in that moment that I had met an angel. I would be forever grateful. From that day forward, I became consciously aware of, and grateful for, the power of strangers in our lives.

Call them angels or compassionate beings, I do believe they demonstrate the power of the Divine in our lives. St. Paul says: "Some have entertained angels unaware." On that day, one of the saddest days of my life, help came my way. I was blessed and I was not alone.

What I have learned from this is that even our simplest actions—smiling to a stranger walking past us on the street, holding the door for someone at the bookstore, or extending a hand to help an elderly person step down a flight of stairs—make a huge difference. When we reach out with gratitude and kindness, remembering the kindnesses bestowed us, well, there are no words to describe how good we feel. And how we know we are never alone.

GRATITUDE PRACTICE

Create gratitude prayer prompters. Incorporate gratitude prayers into your life by using common sensory information from daily life as a trigger to remind you to be grateful for what is right in front of you. Each time you come across these visuals, remind yourself to halt your thoughts for a minute and say a prayer of intentional thanksgiving. Here are some examples:

When you see a fire truck or an ambulance: say thank you for the men and women who are there to take care of the sick and hurting.

When you see a police car: pray for those whose lives are in trouble and give thanks for those who serve, counsel, and protect.

When you see a school bus: give thanks for children everywhere. Pray for our children and pray for the children worldwide who will never have the opportunities we have.

When you pass a church, remember your blessings. Then pray for those in need or those who don't have the grounding and blessings of faith.

BLESSINGS TO CALL ON: TOOLS FOR GRATITUDE AS A SPIRITUAL PRACTICE

Looking for ways to tap into the spiritual power of gratitude? Here, Gahl Eden Sasson, *a spiritual teacher and author of* Cosmic Navigator: Design Your Destiny with Astrology and Kabbalah, *shares tools for committing to the spiritual awakening of the power of gratitude in our lives.*

Om Mani Padme Hum is an old Buddhist prayer designed to invoke compassion and unconditioned love. It is a prayer we can call on to help us tap into gratitude in our lives.

In Tibet they write this mantra on prayer wheels and spin them continuously. These prayer spheres resemble the 10 spheres of the Tree of Life and work in a similar way.

The meaning of this prayer is very profound. It translates to "The Jewel is in the Lotus." The Lotus is a flower that grows in water (the symbol of compassion in Kabbalah as well as Buddhism) out of the mud and dirt. From the darkest and most hidden places the perfect flower emerges.

The Jewel is the pearl. The story of the pearl is the story of the transformation of imperfections and disabilities into a wondrous jewel. The pearl is created when a piece of grit, dirt, or sand is caught in the oyster. The oyster, being another profound symbol of compassion, does not discard the piece of dirt nor does it throw it away as we humans do with our garbage and dirt. The oyster caresses it with a white veil. Like a silent kiss, it embraces the dirt, investing in it love and kindness. Slowly, with patience, the piece of worthless dirt becomes a precious pearl.

The oyster teaches us that we need imperfection (the dirt) to create perfection (the pearl). We should treat our imperfections and disabilities the same way the oyster treats the grain of sand. It simply accepts it.

Kabbalah in Hebrew means "to accept." Kabbalah teaches us how to flow with God's work by accepting it. The oyster holds that same secret; it teaches us to accept our weaknesses and disabilities. We are perfect in our imperfections; that is the secret paradox of life. What makes us perfect is the ability to grow, and we can only grow if we are not yet perfect. As long as we have some imperfections, we are participating in God's creation.

That is the key of life and that is the Jewel in the Lotus. We often spend too much time in gratitude for what is going well in our life, but as God is One, the perfect and imperfect in you are also one. Spend some time focusing on showing your gratitude toward the imperfections that make you so perfect.

GRATITUDE PRACTICE

Practice this Guided Meditation. Spend some moments and think about your own life. In what areas of your life are you challenged by an imperfection, a disability, a block, or something seemingly as small as a piece of sand? Instead of trying to throw it away, destroy it, curse it, label it, or deny it, try to accept and love it. It will be transformed like magic from your inner enemy to your inner guide; from your imperfection to your perfection; from your disability to your Jewel.

Breathe in three times. Imagine that you are breathing in your imperfections. Now breathe out three times. Imagine that you are breathing out your perfections. Between breaths, spend a few seconds imagining your gratitude for everything that you are ascending to the skies and surrounding the world as the oyster's shell surrounds the pearl. May all your challenges be transformed into pearls. Amen.

TOOLS OF THE GRATITUDE TRADE

CARRY YOUR SPIRIT IN YOUR POCKET

You can buy these at stores, or you can create them. Some gift shops and bookstores sell pebbles or smooth river rocks that have positive words scrawled on them: compassion; gratitude; love; thankfulness. If you can't find them, pick up some stones on your next hike and write these words on them with paint pens. Keep them in your pocket, purse, or anywhere you can hold them and know you are carrying your spirit words. At times throughout the day, touch them, and remember to bless yourself and to say thank you and give blessings to others.

CREATE YOUR OWN PRAYER BOOK

Cut out pictures from nature magazines of inspirational or spiritual scenes, and paste them in a spiral notebook. Then add quotes and prayers to create your own inspirational prayer book. Leafing through it can remind you of what you are grateful for and remind you to give thanks in prayer.

CHAPTER FOUR
PRACTICING GRATITUDE IN EVERYDAY LIFE

There are only two ways to live your life. One is as though nothing is a miracle. The other is as though everything is a miracle.

—Albert Einstein

Have you ever made a wish for happiness when blowing out your birthday cake candles? Instead of making a wish for what you don't have, or what you want, stop and think about what you do have and what you are grateful for. You'll find yourself appreciating your home, even though it needs work; your significant other, even though he or she is lacking in any number of qualities; and your day-to-day life.

We all have moments in our lives that are cause for big celebrations and thank-yous—birthdays, graduations, holidays, a new baby being born, or a job promotion. It is easy to pull out the Champagne, light the candles on the cake, and go all out in celebration. But it is embracing the joyful simplicities of every day and discovering their simple delights that are the essence of life. We need to find joy, to be thankful for the everyday moments that bring us comfort and well-being.

All it takes is a shift in our thinking, a mindfulness to focus on what makes us glad to be alive. So, the next time you're driving, your mind full of tasks, take a look at the people strolling on the street. Notice the ones who have smiles on their faces. Those folks are enjoying their walk; they're appreciating the scenery. There is no more profound advice than "stop and smell the roses."

FINDING GRATITUDE
IN THE SIMPLICITY OF LIFE

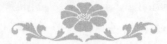

> Who does not thank for little will not thank for much.
>
> —Estonian proverb

Did your parents tell you when you were growing up that "the best things in life are free"? Perhaps they were thinking of the 1927 song by that name that was later recorded by Frank Sinatra and Dinah Shore.

The song's lyrics tell us that "the moon belongs to everyone—the best things in life are free." It takes so little, and costs absolutely nothing, to enjoy—and be grateful for—the scenery all around us.

In this story, Steve Hueston, a high-tech professional and busy single father of two girls, describes a transcendent moment when he took time out at the risk of being *late to work to watch the snow fall.*

In his reverie, he connected the past with the present, and in that moment, reveled in the emotions that have brought him profound pleasure and gratitude.

Steve Hueston was driving his kids to school as another in a series of southwestern Ontario snowstorms started picking up momentum. It was a big one, and, as he tells it, "It was upon us."

This being mid-January, many (although not all—not he, for instance) of what he calls his more efficient neighbors had stripped the decorations from their Christmas trees, boxed up the lights, and set their trees out by the curbside for pickup: just one of the signs of the season.

But this morning he noticed something curious. Whereas a few days before, noticing several trees lying flat by the curb, he had made a mental note to take down his tree as well, on this day he observed that many of them were standing upright, stuck into snowbanks.

"I don't know why this was—maybe folks with a delightful sense of whimsy, maybe testy snowplow operators," Steve says. "The effect, though, was striking. Without the falling snow, it would have been merely fanciful, and would have made me smile. But with the white stuff piling up fast on the branches and thick needles, it was…magical."

He was still thinking about it when he pulled into his

spot at the commuter lot to catch the train into Toronto. Despite the crawling traffic, he was early, so he shut the engine off and watched the snow piling up on the windshield as he reflected on the unexpected Christmas tree forest, and the falling snow—and other things.

"I was struck by powerful feelings of gratitude for all the things—simple, like snow, or the color of the autumn leaves, and not so simple—that have been put in my way, again and again, over and over, for as long as I've been alive," says Steve. "What started out as woolgathering while I waited for my train turned into a rich and almost kaleidoscopic reverie as vignette after vignette faded in and out of view. And the snow kept piling up."

The thoughts of gratitude led him into deep reflection about his own childhood, growing up in Algonquin Park—an immense and fabulous wildlife, camping, and canoeing paradise a couple of hours north of Toronto.

"My dad was the superintendent, so we had a year-round house there, and access to every remote corner or untraveled river, and our summers—and springs, falls, and winters—were spent tasting from the most extraordinary banquet of natural beauty conceivable," he says.

"I'm a pilot now, and every autumn when the leaves change color, I fly up there and just...wander the sky, flying over our old house, our lake (every inch of which I know like the back of my hand), our old canoe routes, and whichever other of our many old haunts I feel like seeing that day. It's always, for one thing, astonishingly beautiful—the spectacle of the gold and red leaves really has to be seen to be believed—but emotional, too (especially now that my dad's gone)—and always leaves me overwhelmed with the rich bounty that's been conferred upon me. Invariably, when I return from these little jaunts, I'm very quiet and thoughtful for a few days—and what's always uppermost in my mind is how grateful I am to have lived the life I have.

"We take these things for granted—but we don't have to. And I find it impossible to experience these things and not feel grateful for whatever magic or divinity put them there for us."

GRATITUDE PRACTICE

Go for a walk and take in the bounty of nature. Look, really look, at the miracle of trees, plants, birds, and insects. As Steve Hueston says, "The really remarkable thing about that moment of clarity was how powerfully it's stayed with me, every day since. I cannot—cannot— hear the wind in the trees, or see the sparkle of sun on water, or watch a waterfall cascading, without stopping to soak it in, and to give thanks. The northern lights! Have you ever seen the northern lights? I defy anyone to watch that insane splendor and not feel tiny and grateful."

SHIFTING GEARS: LEAVING FUNKYTOWN AND GEARING UP TO GRATITUDE

I merely took the energy it takes to pout and wrote some blues.

—Duke Ellington

Tired? Exhausted? Stretched to the max? That seems to be the mantra these days in what appears more like an epidemic of exhaustion than fully living.

The good news? There's a solution: gratitude.

Here, John Duffy shares a snapshot from his very full life, during an "off day." Determined not to walk through his days like a zombie, Duffy decided to take steps to change his perceptions, and in doing so, found himself dragging a little less, and setting happiness and health as his primary goals.

The message: get proactive about your gratitude atti-

tude, and you too can defend yourself against the blues and
other bothersome feelings that block you from fully living
and appreciating the rich moments that appear every day.

John Duffy, a psychotherapist in La Grange, Illinois, describes how last February he found himself in what they call a "bit of a funk."

"I felt sluggish, exhausted really, and slightly under the weather," he says. "I felt a little blue. I was dragging my feet. I was definitely not entirely present, so I knew I was missing moments, probably important ones."

John recalls how he had spent the prior weekend skiing with families from his neighborhood. What should have been fun instead was a blur. "It had its moments, but overall was a blur," he recalls. "The day before, I went to the funeral of a close family friend. I should have been fully present, aware, in the moment. But really, I wasn't. Mostly, I was blah-ish."

John remembers asking himself, This is all circumstantial, right? Winter blues, cabin fever, stuff like that. It'll pass with time. Yep. Just need to give it time. Or am I dealing with something more insidious? Is this malaise a choice I'm making? Is this something I should just be able to "shake"? Is there something in my thinking that "causes" this state of mind, body, and spirit?

But even as he asked himself these questions, he says he already knew the answer.

"Typically, we are unaware of it, but thoughts, all of them, are choices," he says. "If we bring our thoughts into the realm of conscious awareness, we can usually do a more than adequate job of 'diagnosing' the issue or issues that take us out of the game. We can then think about how we think. Do we tend to focus on the negative, the foreboding, and the stressful? Yeah, then we're going to find ourselves out of the game more often than not."

But wait, he remembers thinking. If he could ask himself those questions, he knew he should be able to give himself the self-exam.

"Ta-da. A little self-exam, and I have righted my world," John says. "Sweet."

But he realized that his world still felt fuzzy, dim. "No, see, what I had to do is to think something different." He needed a little redo of his initial thoughts.

So he revised his thoughts about that weekend. "I had the good fortune to ski this weekend. Even with a body a bit under the weather, even with the economy in the shape it's in, I skied. I breathed in the fresh, cool northern Michigan air on a nearly perfect ski day. I watched my wife master the chair lift with delight. I marveled at my son's strength and ease on the hills, and heard the unabated joy of his laughter with his sweet friends.

"And I had the privilege this weekend of honoring the memory of a remarkable woman. Marlene Scholl was not a constant presence in my life, but she made me feel good when we were together. The limitless generosity of her family afforded me the opportunity to go to grad school as a new father strapped for cash. Without them, I would not be seeing my clients today. I would not have the tools to help the people I help today.

"And Marlene suffered far too long. I surely believe she is resting in quiet, gentle peace. And in a strange way, I am grateful for that. And I pray for better, easier days for her husband, Bob, and her extended family."

Maybe a shift in perspective and a little gratitude can go a long way, John's experience showed him.

Just knowing that, he says he felt better almost immediately.

GRATITUDE PRACTICE
When you are feeling blue, write down the feelings you are experiencing and then write down the ones you wish you felt. You'll be so amazed by looking at what comes forward in your writing. It will help you see the blessings in your everyday life.

LISTENING FROM THE HEART: SIMPLE PRACTICES CAN RECONNECT US WITH THE FLOW OF LIFE

Your diamonds are not in far distant mountains or in yonder seas; they are in your own backyard, if you but dig for them.

—Russell H. Conwell

The simple moments, when life shows us its blessings, can be empowering ones. Here, Anne Lee, of Barrington, Illinois, shares a transformative moment when her dear friend Elizabeth phoned, showing Anne that listening is a process of love, free of judgment or expectation.

When we acknowledge what we've learned from others, it helps us all to appreciate the abundance in our lives. Sometimes, it also helps us tap into the positive qualities we embody. Gratitude attracts more gratitude, and opens the gates of tenderness. Anyone who knows Anne Lee knows she is the first to reach out in the midst of fear and uncertainty to listen, care, and be present.

* * *

The phone rang. It was Elizabeth, Anne Lee's close friend with whom she "talks life."

"Hi, Anne, I just called to listen," Elizabeth told her. "Today is National Listening Day—just heard it on NPR. Since you are the best listener I know, I want to give *you* the gift of listening. So, I am here as your friend today to listen to whatever is on your mind or in your heart.

And Elizabeth listened. Across the thousand miles that separated the best friends, Elizabeth was reaching out and connecting.

"I could feel Elizabeth listening," Anne remembers, "and I was grateful. How good it feels to connect and talk about 'questions that matter.' We honor and celebrate one another's lives through listening, really listening."

Through Elizabeth's calling and listening, Anne says her feelings were validated. "She made me feel that I mattered. It felt good. It truly was a gratitude moment!"

Elizabeth explained that the way the Native American listens is to be in total silence, with no responses such as "uh-huh" or "oh," no comments, just listening, hearing, and caring. "Eye to eye, heart to heart, there for each other, that's how they listen."

"Yes, we do carry each other, support one another, and listen to what matters," Anne says. "During that phone call across almost a thousand miles, I felt connected, cared about, and grateful for the friendship. Yes, gratitude grows the spirit."

GRATITUDE PRACTICE

Stop for a moment and be thankful for the giver behind the gift. Make a list of the people in your life who made you happy today. It could be anyone—the clerk at the grocery store who knows you and took the extra time to ask how you and your loved ones were doing, the neighbor who shoveled your sidewalk, or the friend who called unexpectedly just to say she cared. Practicing gratitude is about being thankful for all the blessings in your life—the abundance found in every day.

TURNING THE DAILY COMMUTE INTO
A GRATITUDE WORKOUT

God is in the details.
—Ludwig Mies van der Rohe

Creating a sacred space where we can celebrate our thankfulness is not something we often think of doing. But thanks to Lindsey Rodarmer, we learn here that we need to carve out time, energy, and intention to simply experience and bring forth our feelings of gratitude for what we are and what we have in our lives.

At first, this may be just another "must-do" on our already packed daily agendas. But if we make the time for gratitude, we will soon learn that grace is available to each of us at every moment of every day. We just need to be more purposeful about being present in our "great-full" hearts.

Lindsey and Ryan Rodarmer, newlyweds in Grand Rapids, Michigan, both have very busy, stressful jobs in the publishing industry. And they both moonlight to pay the bills and try to get ahead. To save gas and cash, the couple carpool to work.

"We both have master's degrees and wonder why it seems so difficult to ever get ahead," Lindsey says. "Especially when we were promised for so long that if you go to school, you won't have to worry. Now it seems everyone is worrying. For our part, we often feel like there is no light at the end of the tunnel in this economy."

But, she adds, they hear about friends who have lost their jobs and are struggling to provide for themselves and their small children. "These people would do anything to find some kind of work," says Lindsey. "This past weekend, we even heard about a man who had to move from Michigan to Wyoming for work, leaving his wife and twin daughters behind. They can't even see each other because it's too costly for him to travel back and forth."

To weather an economic downturn that has gripped seemingly everyone they know with fear, Lindsey and Steve are taking advantage of their commute time to transform it into moments to give thanks during these rough times.

"Our goal is to try to take time during those car rides when we could be stressing to be grateful for what we have and to remember not to complain about being so busy,"

Lindsey says. "Because we know some people would give anything to be busy right now and can't find work."

Instead of focusing on why everyone seems so unhappy, the couple is learning to live in the present moment, and to give thanks for that opportunity, as part of their path to joy.

"We also try to take dinnertime together, even if it's just a half hour and frozen stir-fry or hot dogs, to reconnect as often as we can—not work or e-mail, we don't answer the phone, just be with each other and be grateful for having that time together," says Lindsey. "A simple half hour is helping us get through the tough times."

The lessons of gratitude in the couple's life are powerful. To keep that deep awareness at the front of her mind all day long, Lindsay has created a "gratitude list" that hangs in her office. It includes the top 10 things she is grateful for. "Whenever I get down at work, I look at this and remind myself why I am here and why I am so lucky."

Here is the list that allows Lindsey to look beyond the fear and worry of the present economic crisis, and remind herself that she has much for which to be grateful:

1. Braiden is healthy and happy. [Braiden is Lindsey's stepson.]

2. Our health, especially Ryan's health. [Lindsey's husband, Ryan, recovered from a dangerous heart infection.]

3. Marrying for true love, not money, and knowing deep down that we would be happy together, even if we had to give up everything we owned and live in poverty.

4. A safe place to live and food to eat.

5. Our family and friends—so many wonderful people that we hang out with not just because we have to, but we want to.

6. Our jobs (all four of them!).

7. Having the opportunity to teach and shape young minds, and continue learning right along with them. [Lindsey teaches adjunct college courses.]

8. Our dog, which is forever happy to see us and never complains.

9. We get to go on vacation this summer as a family— remember to save money all year for that one glorious week—pay cash, no debt from this vacation.

10. Sharing faith, hope, and trust that things are out of our control anyway, so why not make the best of what we can and live each day as positively as possible.

GRATITUDE PRACTICE

Create a Top 10 list of the things you are most grateful for in your life. Carry it with you in your purse or pocket, or post it on your mirror, your refrigerator, or at your office to remind you daily of what you are grateful for. What you are grateful for will seemingly leap off the page at the times when you most need the reminder.

A MOMENT OF GRACE GIVES WAY
TO A LIFETIME OF GRATEFULNESS

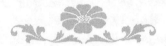

Gratefulness is the key to a happy life that we hold in our hands, because if we are not grateful, then no matter how much we have we will not be happy—because we will always want to have something else or something more.

—Brother David Steindl-Rast

When we wake up each day and live from a starting point of gratitude, no matter what our circumstances might be, feeling grateful or appreciative of someone or something actually attracts more of the things that we appreciate.

Irina Lazar knows this firsthand. What friends have labeled as her "luck" is actually her intention to live each day in thanksgiving and always to live as if good will come. It is that intentional awareness and focus that she believes draws the universe's gifts to her.

* * *

Irina Lazar remembers experiencing a bolt from the blue at the age of 15 while going through a routine activity. She was standing in her closet trying to find something to wear.

"I had a difficult childhood, not because of abuse or neglect, just a hopelessness that followed me around like a little dark cloud," she recalls. "I couldn't tell you the source of that sadness. But as I was standing in my closet, I had a moment when I suddenly felt the veil of sadness lift off of me. I felt that I could do and be anything I wanted. I felt empowered, confident, and most of all, happy."

She wasn't able to discern at that age what it meant; she just felt excited. "My life opened up, I felt alive and ready to take on any opportunity."

That was 17 years ago. Now that Irina is in her thirties, she has reflected a lot on that moment and is grateful. She credits that state of grace to an awareness of gratitude.

"I feel appreciation in my cells every minute of every day," says Irina. "It is the fuel that pulsates through me, driving me to enjoy everything in life, even mundane things like washing dishes, paying bills, and running errands."

Her friends attribute her exciting life to "luck."

Both on and off the job, Irina is grateful for her many life blessings. As a TV producer, she has seen the world. Her travels have taken her to places like Hawaii, Europe, Asia, and South America, and she has lived in New York,

San Francisco, and Los Angeles, which she says are "more like temples than simple places to rest my head." She has worked with some of the most notable and talented musicians, actors, and artists in the world.

"I have a large circle of loving, beautiful, and caring friends," Irina says. "I have parents who love me unconditionally, and even though they may not understand me, they leave their hearts open to me. My life is full of riches."

So is she lucky?

Robert Emmons, a professor of psychology at the University of California, Davis, has conducted numerous research projects with Mike McCullough, a psychology professor at the University of Miami, that are designed to generate scientific data on the nature of gratitude, its causes, and its potential consequences for human health and well-being. Emmons has found that people like Irina Lazar who find something to appreciate every day are less depressed, envious, and anxious and much more likely to help others. Their studies determined that people who count their blessings are happier, healthier, and more likely to achieve their personal goals.

In one study, the professors assigned three groups of volunteers one topic each to focus on for the week. One group focused on grateful thinking, another focused on hassles and irritations, and the third group simply recorded events. They found that a daily gratitude intervention resulted in higher reported levels of the positive states of alertness, enthusiasm, determination, attentiveness, and energy compared to a focus on hassles and irritations.

Irina describes herself as alert: "I am awake to the endless possibilities this life has to offer," she says. "When you are fully awake, colors take on new meaning, little things that you passed by before seem to have new life, and you notice things that you didn't notice before. The early-morning alarm means being able to enjoy more sunshine in the day, being stuck in traffic means more time to relax and breathe, and little annoyances become amusing rather than burdensome."

Living in gratitude has become a joyful challenge that Irina says she likes to make into a game of sorts. She asks for things and then waits to see how they magically appear. For instance, she recently had two experiences that illustrate how "being present gives you presents."

"Last night I said to myself that I needed a new caddy in my shower and a yoga class I could attend once a week," she recalls. "I decided to take advantage of the beautiful day and go for a hike. As I parked the car, I saw that someone had left some free things out in front of their home, and of course there was a shower caddy in perfect condition sitting there waiting for me. I acknowledged this as the universe working in my favor and loaded it into my car. As I approached the entrance to the trail, I saw a yoga class taking place in the field and a sign that read 'Free yoga every day, 10:30–11:45 A.M.' "

Do you see the difference between being lucky and being awake? Irina noticed the opportunities because she is present: she notices what is going on around her. And she projects an optimism and thankfulness for her ability to be present and awake and to love every moment of every day.

GRATITUDE PRACTICE
Using any of the gratitude practices throughout this book, shift into a state of gratitude. Then make a wish, and see if it comes true!

LIGHT A VIRTUAL CANDLE

Light a candle with the intention of saying thanks for what you are grateful for in your life. If you don't have a candle handy, or are not in a place where that is practical, go to http://www.gratefulness.org/candles/enter.cfm?l=eng and you can light a candle in solidarity with others who have found their way to Brother David Steindl-Rast's gratefulness community. Gratefulness.org is a nonprofit organization dedicated to gratefulness as a universal principle that serves as the core inspiration for personal growth, cross-cultural understanding, interfaith dialogue, intergenerational respect, and ecological sustainability.

MUST LOVE DOGS—
MAN'S BEST FRIEND TAKES US BACK TO THE
BASICS OF THANKSGIVING

We can thank our lucky stars when once in a blue moon we find rare and kindred souls along the pathway of our lives.

—Laurel Burch

The people around us aren't our only reminders of the universe's gifts to us in everyday moments. Our daily lives are filled with moments that bring us joy. We just need to learn to savor those small, authentic moments that bring contentment.

Here Diana Rohini LaVigne helps us pause to see the joy we might find in petting our dog, or sipping that first morning coffee, or creating a new culinary experience for dinner. As she shares her discovery of the delight she experiences with her two dogs, it reminds us all to look closer to recognize and embrace moments of happiness

that are uniquely our own, and to give thanks for those
blessings.

Diana Rohini LaVigne and her husband, Vikramaditya
Gupta, are grateful every day for the love and appreciation
their two dogs give them, regardless of anything happening
that day or in the world.

"Just the simple exercise of greeting us at the door can
make any bad traffic on the drive home or a tough day at
work or word of bad news about a loved one vanish for a
few moments," says Diana. The dogs, a seven-year-old pug
named Indy and an eight-year-old pug named Maximus,
give the Fremont, California, couple a daily dose of *shanti*
(peace) that they say keeps them going.

"When we are upset, they know and cuddle us closely
while begging us with their eyes to be happy and celebrate
life," says Diana, who is the head of global communica-
tions for Nair and Co.

Diana confides that people have chided them for the
extraordinary care they give to their canine friends/family
members, but the couple are in agreement that the dogs
give them constant cause for joy and celebration.

"Their love is unconditional, and we love every moment
spent with them," she says. "We express our gratitude
in our level of commitment to our dogs. When we were
looking to buy a house, our dogs and their happiness in
the home were a top priority. We brought them to see our

current home before making a bid. Our dogs helped us buy our home!"

Indeed, the two pugs play a key role in the couple's life, even to the point where they come home early at night so the dogs aren't left alone too long. Additionally, they book 90 percent of their travel with the canines in mind.

"When our dogs are sick, one of us will work from home," Diana says. "On weekends, we try to spend as much time as possible with our dogs. We know all the dog-friendly places and take them with us wherever possible. Restaurants with outside seating, dog-friendly shops, and lazy days at the park are part of our weekly ritual. And our friends are always introduced to our dogs as though they are family members. It makes a difference, as I've seen others treat my dogs like children, not like pets, because of our high regard for our dogs. It helps that they are also a highly friendly breed, I'm sure. But when we go to the vet or dog park, everyone remembers my dogs' names, not ours, necessarily."

Diana is proof of the stress reduction dogs can bring, and she is thankful for the respite from her busy work life they provide. "I am a workaholic by nature, and yet watching them play is one of the few things that relax me enough to take a real break."

GRATITUDE PRACTICE

If you have a pet, take a few moments to list the blessings your beloved animal brings to your life. Perhaps your cat keeps your toes warm at night. Or give thanks that because of your dog you get outside every day for exercise. Give thanks for the unconditional love of your pet.

GETTING INTO THE HABIT OF APPRECIATION AND GRATITUDE FOR YOUR TEEN

The transformation from tween to teen can be a hard one—not only for the young person, but for the parents. The dreaded phase "the terrible twos" has shifted to "the terrible teens." To help change your thinking and find the blessing in these years of transformation for your child, Dr. John Duffy offers this meditation exercise.

Find a time when your teenager is occupied in a more public area of your home, somewhere other than her bedroom. She may be reading, talking on the phone, playing a game, or listening to music. For the purposes of this exercise, as long as she is occupied, it really doesn't matter what she is doing.

Now find a comfortable seat in another room. First, gently remove from your mind, just for these moments, any feelings of anger, ill will, disappointment, or resentment you harbor toward her. Take a few moments alone to close your eyes and take a few deep, cleansing breaths. For the next several minutes, assume that all is right with the world. You needn't worry about a thing. You can cast all of your concern, just for now, totally aside.

As you inhale, allow your lungs to fill with a sense of well-being and contentment. As you exhale, envision your negative thoughts leaving you. Once you feel calm, open your eyes. Stand up and take a seat in the room where you child is occupied. Continue your deep breathing.

Just watch her discreetly for a few moments as you attend to your breathing. Sit quietly, watch and listen. With no demand on yourself, take note in your mind of what you see in her, what you hear from her. Look at the shine of her hair. Allow yourself to marvel at the perfection of her hands. Listen to her voice and her laughter, her very breathing. Watch her smile. Does she ponder her world? In what ways does she look like you? Now look at your child's beautiful eyes. How long has it been since you have seen them in this way? Breathe in the miracle that is your teenager.

When you feel ready, go back to the room where you began this exercise, relaxing and breathing. Have a seat, and take a few more cleansing breaths. Think about your teenager. How are you feeling about her now?

In this exercise, Dr. Duffy says he is encouraging parents to see their teenager with the same sense of wonder they felt when they first laid eyes on her, when she was a newborn baby. Parents who have participated fully in this exercise will feel "pretty wonderful," he says.

"If you conduct this exercise from time to time, you

may find you get in the habit of appreciation and gratitude for the presence of your teenager in your life," Dr. Duffy says. "She makes things interesting, doesn't she? She is a force. She can be upsetting and frustrating, yes. This in fact is part of her job. At her core, though, underneath it all, she is wonderful and amazing—a miracle, really."

Through this exercise Dr. Duffy encourages parents to see themselves as fortunate. "You have the opportunity to parent this wonderful, challenging person, to affect the future of her life, your life, your family, and perhaps everyone. A large responsibility, yes, but none could equal the rewards of parenting."

CHAPTER FIVE
STAYING THANKFUL IN DIFFICULT TIMES

Something opens our wings.
Something makes boredom and hurt disappear.
Someone fills the cup in front of us.
We taste only sacredness.

—*Rumi*

No one wants to endure heartache or suffering. None of us would voluntarily choose to lose our jobs, see our family members struck down by illness, or have a cherished relationship end. But it is often after these times of difficulty, heartache, and anguish that blessings come.

Many believe that strength only comes through struggle. It is a common refrain that what doesn't kill us makes us stronger. Ironically, many of us find we become more compassionate, more caring, and better people after we have moved through difficulties or periods of trauma.

In this chapter, we are inspired by the creative ways

people facing difficult times have dug beneath the surface to uncover what they are grateful for. They help us find ways to articulate our thankfulness and remind us that no matter what challenges we face in life, rainbows follow clouds and rain.

ZEN HABITS:
LIVING WITH THANKSGIVING
CAN CHANGE YOURLIFE

Gratitude is a vaccine, an antitoxin, and an antiseptic.

—John Henry Towett

Every day is a good day to practice gratitude. Just ask Jenny Runkel, who, after being diagnosed with lymphoma at age 32, decided to put her heart into all things thankful— her husband, her two young children, and inspiring others. Her mantra comes from Virgil: "They can conquer who believe they can."

We share Jenny's story here because we believe gratitude helps heal body, mind, and soul. Through Jenny's story, we hope you too will know that gratitude can unlock the fullness in your life and create a new vision for tomorrow, no matter how difficult today may seem.

* * *

"I just practiced yoga for the first time today," Jenny reports. "I mean, I have done yoga many times before, but this time was markedly different. In the past, yoga has been a part of my routine. My workout. Another 'thing to do' that I check off of my list so that I could get on to other, more important matters. In fact, I used to see it as an 'off' day in my schedule of working out."

But that was before cancer swooped in and invaded her body.

Before that, her idea of exercise was aerobic activity that left her sweating and exhausted.

"I felt like I didn't really work out unless it was for an hour at a time and I really smelled bad once I was finished," Jenny says. "Because of that mentality, I never really enjoyed my time with myself. I was always pressing, always feeling like I didn't measure up if I didn't push harder or go further. What I failed to notice was how good it felt when I was doing it—any of it."

It's amazing how a little thing like a tumor can change all that.

Before this "journey," she says she used to worry about finding the time to fit in five workouts a week. "And, trust me, they had to be workouts."

But cancer brought her a new appreciation of what exercise and taking care of herself means.

"Now, for the first time, I feel differently about my

body and the way it works," she says. "I don't feel like I'm fighting against it, trying to win some battle of the bulge. It isn't an adversary, standing in the way of happiness and a perfect size six. Instead, it is my friend. It is trying so hard to get rid of this stuff, and exercise means something totally different."

The first thing Jenny feels like doing when she wakes up is yoga.

It has become her lifeline and the healing force she is ever so grateful for.

"Not because I had to, or because that is what my routine dictated," she says. "I felt like doing it because I felt good. And when I did it, it made me feel even better. All the cheesy little phrases they say on the video (that I never paid attention to before) suddenly felt like real nuggets of wisdom. This time, I wasn't rushing through the poses or seeing how fast I could move from one to another. Instead, I was luxuriating in the fact that I could lift my arms straight up above my head without that annoying pull of Steri-Strips. (They finally fell off a day or two ago!!)"

Instead of rolling her eyes at the "wisdom" of using your breath to get into or out of a pose, she found herself enjoying the fact that she could take a deep breath over and over again. And when the tape was over, instead of rushing off to jump on the treadmill to finish her workout, she just sat there thinking about the last thing her instructor said: "You see that there is no war within you. You're on your own side, and you are your own strength. Your body becomes a connection between heaven and earth."

So, as Jenny says, "I guess, for today, I'm thankful for yoga. And for what my body can do. And for coffee—because coffee is always good. But don't worry; I'm not going to go hard-core hippie or anything. Unless it really continues to make me feel better. If that's the case, I just might grow out my leg hair and only eat wheatgrass shakes. Who knows?"

Jenny has been in remission for four years.

"My doctor tells me how remarkable my recovery was every time she sees me," says Jenny. "I am the picture of health now and I view exercise much the same way now as I learned to then. I play tennis a couple of times a week to enjoy the fresh air and the friendship of others, and I play outside with my kids every chance I get. I am even thankful for jogging—I am reminded how very hard it was at one point to simply take a deep breath—and now I can run around as much as I want."

Jenny also is dedicated to gratitude in her professional life, as a writer for two websites devoted to helping families enjoy each other and not fight. ScreamFree.com focuses on the relationships between parents and children, and SheJustGotMarried.com focuses on helping newlyweds get off to a good and healthy start.

GRATITUDE PRACTICE

Find a yoga class near you. Experiment as you go through the practice. Be open to whatever happens when you venture out and experiment with yoga as a way to heal body, mind, and spirit. And be grateful for those moments.

SAVED TO SERVE:
FROM PRISONER OF WAR TO THE PULPIT

Give thanks for a little and you will find a lot.
—The Hausa of Nigeria

Sometimes it is in our darkest moments that we need to trust that a power greater than ourselves will help us move out of our despair. How many of us have cried out in despair, "God, please help me?" and then realized that no matter what is taken away, no matter what hurricane rips through your life, you will survive, and you are grateful for everything you have had so far.

In this story, we come to know a man who almost died, a man who was a prisoner of war, suffered countless illnesses, and yet more than 30 years later, has made it his life mission to give thanks for his survival and to help others as a minister. In this story we hold close the words of Eleanor Roosevelt: "You gain strength, courage and confidence by every experience in which you really stop to look fear in the face. You must do the thing you cannot do."

No coward soul is Louis Kerkstra. No trembler in the face of adversity. Growing up on a farm in Michigan as one of 10 children, Louis had an eighth-grade education when he was drafted into the Korean War.

During that war, he was captured and spent two years in a POW camp. While there, he became extremely ill with tuberculosis, dysentery, jaundice, pleurisy, and frostbite. He was very close to death's door.

One night, when his Chinese captors were making their rounds, shining their flashlights into the faces of prisoners to see who had died, Louis remembers an overwhelming feeling that he was going to make it; God had other plans for his life.

After being released in a prisoner exchange and returned to the United States, he spent almost 16 months recuperating in hospitals, followed by a long stint in rehabilitation. From there he went on to college and seminary and has spent the last 32 years as a minister.

But he will never forget the day in 1953 when one of the guards came into his room and said: "Get your things; you are going to go home."

"It seemed as though I was living in a dream too good to be true," recalls Louis.

In "Freedom Village," after two years in captivity, Louis received communion from a chaplain. It was then that he decided to devote his life to helping others out of gratefulness.

These days, Louis spends his days ministering to the sick and suffering.

"I am deeply grateful that I can help others," he says. "I feel blessed to better help others who are suffering and I know it was worth going through the suffering I endured, as I was assured of the Lord's presence and care for me. For that I will be forever grateful."

LOVING A SON TO WHOLENESS: GRATEFUL TO SURVIVE AND SURMOUNT ILLNESS

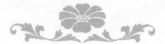

When a person doesn't have gratitude, something is missing in his or her humanity. A person can almost be defined by his or her attitude toward gratitude.

—Elie Wiesel

For many of us, the thought of seeing our child go through adversity is unbearable. We want to take the pain and make it our own.

That is why letting go of the stress, the fear, and the anger is a significant feat. How do we find "the good" when our child is suffering? What is the opportunity? The blessing?

In this story, we are inspired by the gratitude experienced in the highs and lows. In dealing with their son's cancer, one couple learned the power of being grateful during the worst times, and the times when the cancer battle seemed to be won. They inspire us through illness to be grateful for the small hurdles and to take each day as it comes.

Twelve years ago, Finn and Paula Waaramaa got the call. Their son, a college student, was diagnosed with Hodgkin's lymphoma.

"Anyone who has experienced the stages of living through the entire cancer journey understands the gratitude received, mixed in with the extreme lows," says Finn.

He says he will never forget the doctor calling from the University of Arizona Medical Center. "He did not want to say that much over the phone but wanted us to understand his concerns for our son," Finn recalls.

The whole thing happened so fast. Darin, Finn's son, had been home recently for his grandmother's funeral. His mom became concerned with his persistent coughing and insisted that Darin see a doctor.

Then came the call to Finn at work. The doctor said something was showing on the X ray that gave him cause for concern.

"I will always remember communicating to my boss using the white board to write that Darin might have cancer. I could not say the words," Finn says.

"I was freaking out and had to leave work immediately. My wife was out of town visiting a friend and she was not going to hear the news until I got her from the gate at the airport and into the car, sitting down. You can only imagine how I felt when we completed the walk and I got her in a private place. This is her baby. Yes, a college student and our second-born but her baby."

Despite the diagnosis, Darin had a type of cancer that is curable. And very fortunately, says Finn, the family had the medical insurance to cover the treatment. "We thanked our lucky stars," Finn remembers.

"Anytime we hear of someone experiencing problems with medical insurance coverage, well, we are grateful for what we had," he says. "They will never be able to know the difference between drugs that work, although expensive, and other choices being made that are less effective. Oh my God, how lucky my son was that we had fantastic coverage. It was a feeling of gratitude we will take to our graves."

A year after Darin's treatment, cancer invaded again. Again, it was treated and their son was told he was in remission. Even though he remains so, Finn says the family gets anxious after every test, always waiting to make sure the tests are negative, and always grateful they have been.

Finn explains: "We all put our faith in his doctors and they proved to steer us down the correct path. Anyone in their right mind would have expressed the level of gratitude that we felt. Test after test and year after year, we still wait for the all-clear report. And even after twelve years of good news, July and August are not our most favorite months."

Today, Darin and his wife are the proud parents of two children. Their oldest daughter is named Grace. Finn says, "You can only imagine our gratitude, as grandparents, for his life and the joy we share."

GRATITUDE PRACTICE
Start each day with the Modeh Ani—a Jewish morning prayer:

I am thankful before You,
Living and Sustaining Ruler,
Who returned my soul to me with mercy.
Your faithfulness is great.

THE GOOD NEWS:
HONORING DAILY GLIMPSES OF GRATITUDE

It was during one of life's toughest times that Vikki Smith decided she would focus on the good in her life.

So during her divorce from her husband of 27 years, the Austin, Texas, mom of two kids, ages 21 and 23, knew her life was going to change in many ways when her husband moved out.

That is when she began writing every night in a "grateful" journal. "I keep it on my bedside table and before turning out my light each night, I make a point to list something for which I'm grateful," Vicki says. "Some days I have ten things—normally, this is when I manage to get in bed earlier and have more time—and some days I'm exhausted and can only manage to get one or two things written. I do not limit myself and find that sometimes I'm repetitive or very general. I might write that I am grateful for healthy children, a roof over my head, or health insurance."

But she also likes to be more specific to the particular day. "I might write that I am grateful to find the kitchen clean when I returned home from work this evening. (My sons have moved back home while finishing up college.)"

Recently, her entry was this: "I am grateful to find

some little blossoms have pushed through the tangled mess that is my front garden. Despite all my efforts to impede it by my negligence, the garden, too, was determined to be grateful for spring and the opportunity to bloom anew."

It is easy to be disgruntled daily—there will always be challenges that block our way to achieving our goals or desires. Writing in her journal helps Vicki remember that "the true joys in life come from recognizing the gift in each moment—not in the final hour."

IN THE AFTERMATH OF THE HURRICANE: GIVING BACK IN GRATITUDE

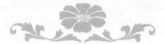

Take full account of the excellencies which you possess, and in gratitude remember how you would hanker after them, if you had them not.

—*Marcus Aurelius*

When adversity hits our lives, sometimes we feel like we have been thrown into a hurricane, spun around, shaken up, and spit back out into the world, stripped of what was before, confused, lost, and afraid about what lies ahead.

Troubled times and new beginnings can be very scary. But for all that we can't control, as we get up off the mat and move back into life there is something we can do that will make all the difference in moving on and starting over: giving thanks for those who carried us through the storm, and those who are there to help us begin again.

When we give thanks to those who have been so kind, an

attitude of gratitude emerges that helps us reenter life and catapults us from the margins of despair to the center of life and rebirth. The following story speaks volumes about the souls of survivors who have weathered adversity and now are giving back in thanks for their new beginnings.

When Hurricane Ike hit the Houston area in September 2008, Ellen Delap could not believe it. Her son, Jake, his two young children, six weeks and three years old, and his wife, Meredith, rushed to her home to "hunker down" and ride out the storm. There, Ellen, her husband, J.Q., and the clan lay awake through the night listening to the wind and rain pelt their home.

When forceful winds took out the electricity in the early morning hours, Ellen's husband and son sprang into action and started the generator. In a haze of sleepiness it occurred to her how thankful she was to have a generator. More grateful thoughts followed: *How thankful that we are all together for this; how thankful I am for preparedness with batteries; how thankful to have an engineer husband who knows how to run a generator.*

Ellen's son and husband stood watch on and off throughout the night. *How grateful I am for protectors of our family*, she remembers thinking. The eye of the storm passed over at 5:30 A.M. with an eerie stillness. *How grateful I am for no damage to our home.* The day dawned with ferocious winds. *How grateful I am for our granddaughter Eva to spend time with and to focus on her rather than the weather.* The ferocious weather continued until the evening, when the storm had passed through. The family ventured outside to inspect the damage. *How grateful that we have our fence standing. How grateful for what little damage.*

In the wake of the storm, when families emerged to scope out the damage, an attitude of gratitude embraced the community. Families focused on relationships and people, not "stuff," Ellen says. Family and friends gathered for shared meals, neighbors met neighbors they had never met before, and children rode bikes rather than cling to their disabled computers and video games.

"Many people realized they were grateful for this return to simplicity even after each community finally got their electricity again," she says.

In the two weeks it took to get the power back, Ellen focused on thankfulness for the little things. "Were we ever grateful for the ability to turn on a hair dryer," she recalls.

They were blessed in the little damage their home received. But more, Ellen and her family felt it was important to express their thankfulness by giving back and helping those less fortunate.

"This gratitude helped us help others who were not as fortunate," she says. "We were able to add support to those most in need this way."

These days, Ellen is committed to giving back to her community. She has helped organize two charities: Mothers Against Cancer, and a fundraising effort for Texas Children's Hospital and Kingwood Women's Club, a group that helps women in the northeastern area of Houston.

Now, Ellen says, "The power of gratitude in my life makes me be a happier 'me' each day. In tough times or everyday life, just by recognizing what is best in my life, I find more joy, more good, and I am a better person to myself and others. This attitude serves me well in affirming those around me I work with, live with, and interact with throughout each day. Most importantly, I consciously set forth this gratitude by thanking those around me daily for big and small things. Being grateful makes all the difference to me."

GRATITUDE PRACTICE
Create a living prayer of thanksgiving by providing a service to a neighbor—shoveling their driveway, mowing their lawn, running an errand, or volunteering with a community organization.

THE MOST IMPORTANT LESSON IN LIFE: IT'S NOT ABOUT THE THINGS

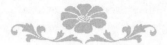

He is a wise man who does not grieve for the things which he has not, but rejoices for those which he has.

—Epictetus

As the saying goes, "A door closes, and a window opens." Those who survive trauma or loss often say it is because they found the fortitude to grieve for their loss, and then push forward to begin again.

Here, we see how after darkness there comes a dawn and a new beginning. Finding gratitude in the unknown, in what lies ahead, can help us shed the burden of the loss in order to clear space for something better to arrive.

A friend phoned Amy LaMae Brewer in a panic. "Come home! We are waiting down the street where you live. Your home is burning."

Amy and her husband rushed back and watched from the other side of the street as flames reached out the windows of their attic while water from the fire hoses tried to tame the conflagration. "We had been remodeling to suit our family of five," Amy says of her home in McMinnville, Oregon. "We had cared for it and given it new life from the day we moved in. It was home."

After three hours and five fire trucks, what remained was a blackened shell. Soaked and damaged, their home could not be recovered. Precious artwork made by the children, antiques and gifts from family, the quilt made by the hands of a beloved grandmother—all lost.

Later, as Amy walked through the darkened debris, she felt the emptiness of things and how these things really were not part of her life anymore. How would we fill a home again with history and loved memoirs? she remembers thinking. "My husband and I held the hands of our children; somehow we all were spared from any harm. In the first days their hands were reminders of thanks each time I held them."

But making sense of this crisis was still difficult for her. It came too fast; the house was gone before plans could be made. "What is the first step in a crisis?—blessings, count the blessings. This is what I learned long ago to do when what you have is little. I did not recognize this at first because I wanted my past blessings back. Still, the blessings came and I began to count."

Climbing out of chaos was difficult but it became a rewarding path for her family.

"Count your blessings—this phrase echoed in my mind," says Amy. "I looked back and realized it began with the child from across the street, in the evening after the fire was put out. A friend to my boys, he raced into his house and said, 'Mom, I need a box!' He returned to the curb with a box full of cars and dinosaurs, the toys he knew my boys liked. 'Here,' he said. 'They can have these toys of mine.' Another neighbor boy came to us with what was in his piggy bank to share with my sons. The parents told us the children gave freely, without any prompting. Amazing gratitude flooded my heart for these dear boys who know what to do in a crisis. Their act of giving produced a gift, a blessing."

Friends and family also rushed to their aid with essentials: toothbrushes, nightclothes, shelter. One mother drove all around town to find a specific sleep toy for one son who needed its comfort. The replaced objects were not the true gift; it was the actions of people giving and the hugs, a clutched hand, a deep sigh, concerned eyes, and men with courage to fight the fire.

"That evening we were touched with the intangible gifts of life that do not fade," Amy says. "People of action fill the well of gratitude."

"We not only had enough for ourselves as mountains of clothes came for my boys, furniture came to our doorstep, quilts came in the mail, and generous people shared what they could; we also could share with others. My children knew that people cared for them. Then this blessing continued. My children knew they not only had friends and people in a community who help when help is needed, they too were able to give from our experience. Thankfulness fills our need and flows over.

"We continued to drink from this well of gratitude in the coming months of redirection and rebuilding," Amy says. "Our town, our church, our family and friends, the neighbors I do not even know, continued to fill our lives and renew our spirits. I cannot go back to my once comforting home, nor do I want to, without the knowledge of such gifts. The truly inspiring power of humanity to care for one another is hope when the walls are gone."

GRATITUDE PRACTICE

Embrace the questions. As you look ahead, ask yourself what you hope to be a year from now. What do you need to live the joyous, creative new life you hope for? What do you need to change? Use this as your mantra:

> *Be patient toward all that is unsolved in your heart and try to love the questions themselves.*
> — *Rainer Maria Rilke*

FINDING THE LIGHT IN DARK DAYS

Sometimes we feel deflated, or overwhelmed, or someone or something hurts us, disappoints us, or we hear bad news about a loved one's medical condition. On those days, when you feel your light has gone out, remember there is always a glimmer of hope and something to be thankful for.

Sometimes our light goes out, but is blown again into instant flame by an encounter with another human being. Each of us owes the deepest thanks to those who have rekindled this inner light.

—Albert Schweitzer

CHAPTER SIX

THE POWER OF GRATITUDE TO MAKE
A DIFFERENCE IN THE WORLD

Happiness is not so much in having as sharing. We make a living by what we get, but we make a life by what we give.

—Norman MacEwan

We are inspired by the people in this chapter who have used their bounty and their spirit of thankfulness to reach out and help others. It doesn't matter what our circumstances are, there is no better way to rise above our circumstances than to volunteer to help a charitable organization, mentor someone, or give counsel and support to someone who needs us. Our thankfulness can manifest itself in our actions and our deeds, in the choice to share our gifts and abundance with those who need it most. And evidence suggests that helping others may be as important to our physical well-being as regular exercise and proper nutrition.

The people in these stories inspire us to embrace giving and to understand that our highest purpose is to give to others. When we do, gratitude becomes contagious—the act of giving thanks and giving back changes the world.

Gratefulness drives out alienation, there is no room in the heart for both. When you are grateful, you say yes to belonging and you reach out to share your gratitude with others through volunteering and putting gratefulness into action. Gratitude strengthens—caring for others is draining, but grateful caregivers are healthier than less grateful ones.

—Brother David Steindl-Rast

NO CHILD LEFT UNFED:
HOW ONE WOMAN FINDS HER SEARCH
FOR MEANING—AND MANY REASONS
TO BE GRATEFUL

Ultimately, man should not ask what the meaning of his life is, but rather must recognize that it is he who is asked. In a word, each man is questioned by life; and he can only answer to life by answering for his own life; to life he can only respond by being responsible.

—*from* Man's Search for Meaning, *by Viktor Frankl*

Karen Sokal-Gutierrez, MD, an associate clinical professor in UC Berkeley and UCSF's Joint Medical Program, and site director for PRIME-US (Program in Medical Education for the Urban Underserved), was deeply affected by Viktor Frankl's book Man's Search for Meaning. *An Austrian psychiatrist and Holocaust survivor, Frankl wrote that even after suffering the barbarity of concentration camps, one still has a chance to find meaning in life.*

For Karen, that meant finding a way to make a difference in the world. She has been drawn to address one of the biggest health issues worldwide, childhood malnutrition. Through Karen's volunteer collaboration with the Salvadoran Association for Rural Health, childhood malnutrition has been dramatically reduced in a region of El Salvador. Karen is now working to bring the program to other Latin American countries.

In this story, Karen fills us in on her groundbreaking work and how grateful she is for finding fulfillment and meaning by doing good.

Karen Sokal-Gutierrez grew up in a comfortable middle-class suburban family. Beginning in childhood, she knew that she'd strive for a fulfilling career, inspired by her family's tradition of working women, including her mother, who is an editor, and her grandmother, who was a doctor.

After graduating from Yale University, Karen spent two years serving in the Peace Corps in rural Ecuador, working in community health and development. She says, "It opened my eyes to the way that the majority of the people in the world live in poverty and poor health, and focused my resolve to make a difference in the world." Motivated to become a physician, she completed medical school at the University of California, San Francisco, trained in pediatrics at Children's Hospital Oakland, and received her master's in public health from UC Berkeley.

She got married, had two children, and settled into her medical career and family routines in Piedmont, California. For a while, Karen found herself consumed with the day-to-day responsibilities of work and family. But, she recalls, "Questions kept nagging at me. *Is this all that there is? How can I make a difference in the world?*"

Ten years later, she was drawn back to Latin America, where she did public health consulting in Guatemala. She found this very rewarding until her group was held up at machine gunpoint by a paramilitary squad. In the moments of terror, she found herself bargaining with God that if she were let off alive, she would stay safely at home.

But after 10 more years at home, she looked for something that could give her life deeper meaning. In 2000, Karen decided to go to El Salvador for a week to volunteer for a nonprofit, nongovernmental rural health organization, *Asociación Salvadoreña Pro-Salud Rural* (ASAPROSAR), a local organization dedicated to improving health by educating and "empowering" the people in rural communities.

Each year over the past 10 years, Karen has returned to El Salvador to volunteer and lead a team of volunteers—doctors, dentists, teachers, and students in the fields of medicine, nursing, and public health, and even her daughter Lia, now 18. The volunteers stay in a dormitory in a local hospital, and pay their own way. Karen's focus has been on providing training for ASAPROSAR's community health workers to improve the health of the children, one-third of whom suffer from malnutrition.

In 2003, Karen and one of her medical students noted that the children who greeted them with hugs and smiles had blackened and decayed teeth. When they asked the parents and health workers whether anyone was addressing this issue, the response was, "No, we've never thought of it as a health problem—it's just a fact of life here."

Returning to the U.S., they researched the public health and medical literature and found that the link between tooth decay and childhood malnutrition—and the possibility of reducing malnutrition by reducing tooth decay—had so far been neglected.

So they undertook a study to assess the prevalence, causes, and complications of tooth decay in the young children. They found that 85 percent of the children under seven years of age had tooth decay and half were in constant pain. "Can you imagine?" says Karen. "So many young children in pain—they can't eat, they can't play, they can't sleep." The study found many possible causes—lack of fluoridated water, poor nutrition during pregnancy and childhood, inability to afford toothbrushes, toothpaste, and dental care. Unfortunately, too, the "modern," American-influenced culture of baby bottles, soda, chips, and candy has lured people away from their healthier traditions of breastfeeding and eating tortillas and beans, damaging children's nutrition and health.

Karen presented the study results to the Director of ASAPROSAR, Dr. Vicky Guzman, a pioneering and courageous woman who started the program during El Salvador's civil war. Karen said to her, "If I were to tell you that a certain medical condition affected 85 percent of the children in this region, and half of the children experienced daily pain from this condition, what would you say?" Dr. Guzman responded, "That would be a major epidemic!" To which Karen replied, "Yes, it is an epidemic—an epidemic of tooth decay." Dr. Guzman's response: "I never thought this was a health problem that we could address—but we need to."

Karen hypothesized that the children's malnutrition could be caused by their tooth decay—the chronic infection, continual pain, and rotten teeth which prevented them from eating. The volunteer team and ASAPROSAR decided to develop an intervention to reduce tooth decay and study whether they could also improve the children's nutrition and health. The team has brought nutrition education, toothbrushes and toothpaste, and fluoride varnish to thousands of children, following up every year with exams of the children and interviews of the mothers.

The results to date have been enormously gratifying.

"We've managed to cut tooth decay and malnutrition in half. Now the majority of the children in the villages have healthy teeth, are pain-free, and well-nourished," Karen says. She recalls a conversation with one of the rural Salvadoran mothers who told her, "We thought that there was nothing we could do about our children's rotten teeth, mouth pain, and malnutrition—it was just a fact of life here. But now we know that childhood doesn't have to be a time of suffering, it can be a time of health and happiness."

Karen's story illustrates the many ways we can experience gratitude through the act of giving back. As she tells it, "Through my experiences in El Salvador, I have found many things for which I am grateful. First, I have been able to reconnect with myself. I have learned from poor people about truly appreciating and enjoying the things that don't cost anything—family and friends, telling stories and jokes, playing music, singing and dancing, and being in nature. And I have learned from uneducated people about the value of common sense, and skills that are passed on for generations. Above all, I've had an opportunity to share my own and my colleagues' medical expertise, and our hearts, and to really help improve the health of the children."

"When I return every year and see the children looking healthier and happier, with pudgy pink cheeks and broad smiles with white teeth, my gratitude for being able to make a difference is immeasurable."

HEALING PLANET EARTH

On Earth Day 2008, Karen Talavera, a Palm Beach County, Florida, writer, mom, and marketing professional, remembers asking herself, Wouldn't it be great if we could use gratitude to help create a better Earth? To help heal the catastrophic environmental destruction we've inflicted in merely a century?

So she came up with a powerful proposal.

While there are thousands, if not tens of thousands, of Earth Day events planned worldwide, this is the easiest to participate in, and perhaps the most universal. It's called "10 Minutes of Gratitude for Planet Earth." This is what you do:

On Earth Day, at 12:00 noon in your time zone, sit quietly for 10 minutes and think of all the places, experiences, and moments of Earthly nature you have ever enjoyed, and be grateful for them. This event is not intended to be a simultaneous, central gathering in one place, but will happen everywhere at noon in each time zone. People may certainly gather together in groups if they wish.

Yep, that's it. You don't have to go anywhere, give any money, or receive any solicitations. It's a seemingly simple idea, but think of the chain of gratitude that could be created if everyone took the time to test Karen's idea.

GIVING THANKS FOR THE
OPPORTUNITY TO GIVE

Reaching out to others fuels the collective power of gratitude.

> *It takes a person of great heart to see ... the wisdom the elders have to offer, and so serve them out of gratitude for the life they have passed on to us.*
> —Ken Nerburn

When we were children, many of us were schooled to associate saying "Thank you" with obligation and even guilt. Our parents would say to us, "Say thank you to Grandma for the pajamas" or "When I was a child I had to make my own toys from rocks and sticks, and look at everything you have that you take for granted."

Many of us carried this idea of saying "Thank you" as an obligation into adulthood. These memories can cause us to feel an underlying sense of resentment when we owe someone a thank-you or feel that someone has not sufficiently thanked us. There is a not-so-subtle feeling of obligation.

But, ironically, giving and gratitude often take us by surprise. Often, we find that it is in our own giving that we receive. And when we realize this, we feel so thankful for the shift in ourselves—for the light that comes on in our minds and the surprising sense of well-being we acquire through our giving.

Here, Sherry Zimmerman of Chicago helps us see how giving to others is a gift to ourselves, one we can embrace and be thankful for.

Each week, Sherry Zimmerman volunteers at Little Brothers – Friends of the Elderly. The mission of Little Brothers is to enlist volunteers to bring friendship to elders who live alone or are in nursing homes. In many cases their families live far away, or there are no living relatives or relatives who can care for them; many have outlived their friends and find they are physically unable to get out and find new friends or participate in daily living, like going shopping, to church, and to the places they used to love.

Sherry began her service by writing articles for the organization's Volunteer Newsletter, including a monthly feature titled "An Old Friend Is Waiting" that profiles an elder in need of a visitor.

After a few years, Sherry became a visiting volunteer. The first elder she was assigned to visit was Loretta Bamman, a very petite and alert woman in her eighties who had outlived all but one of her friends and was almost completely blind from macular degeneration. She had one son who lived in another state but was unable to visit her. Loretta was proud that he would call her once a week.

"It surprised me that Loretta was so positive and lived for the moment," Sherry recalls. "She had been a painter, a singer, and a poet. When her vision was nearly gone, she gave away all of her personal belongings except for some clothing, a few paintings, and her books of poetry and then checked herself into a nursing home."

"I had to learn to approach her gently when I visited. It was easy to forget about her blindness because you can't tell by appearance that someone has macular degeneration and can't see you coming. Eventually, the sound of my greeting would make her eyes light up like she was looking right at me."

Loretta told Sherry that her personal appearance was very important to her. Although without sight, she still had the painter's vision and sense of color. She dressed to the nines every day and was never without jewelry. Unfortunately, in the nursing home, an item of clothing that was sent to be washed might not be returned; a different item might come back. This disturbed her.

"She asked me to go through her closet to put outfits that matched on one hanger," Sherry says. "I started visiting thrift stores to find pretty outfits for Loretta. One day I asked her to come with me to shop. I wanted to help restore some sense of the power of personal choice in her life. She had gone from total independence to being at the mercy of the nursing home staff and whatever charity came her way. We arrived at a large Salvation Army type of thrift store. I found an old metal folding chair and parked her at the end of the aisle, bringing her nearly new things to touch and feel, describing the color and pattern. While looking through the racks, I saw little kids running around, bumping into her and the chair and squealing."

Seeing this, Sherry became concerned and thought the adventure was a big mistake. "There she was, blind, probably not comfortable, unknown chaos and activity all around her. I asked if she was okay and was shocked by her response."

"She said, 'Sherry, just think. Here are all these parents who can't afford much at all. They can come here and outfit their entire family for just pennies. Isn't that wonderful?'"

Loretta passed away about five years ago. Sherry says, "It was sad that we were the only ones at her burial besides a lady who was close to her from a church she attended, and the manager of the nursing home. She had made all of the arrangements for herself. I was glad that she suffered very little at the end. Just a couple days in the hospital in ICU with heart failure. Such a special woman. She spoke and lived by the phrase 'My attitude is gratitude.' Loretta was a real joy."

At her burial, Sherry read a couple of Loretta's poems.

As the minister said the final prayer, Sherry thought of another lesson that Loretta had taught her when she said, "I feel that our prayers are stronger when we pray for others."

Today, Sherry is still inspired by Loretta's writings. The poem below, which Loretta wrote in her eighties, underscores the wisdom and depth of soul that she brought to those around her, a gift that Sherry will always be grateful for.

WHAT IS A FRIEND?

When a friend says "I need you!" what do you say?

Do you say "What happened?" or do you say "How can I help?"

Does it really matter what happened—or does it matter only that your friend needs you; has asked for your help

God never asks us—"What happened?"

He says: "I love you—I am your friend!"

For the last five years, since Loretta's death, Sherry has been visiting a new elder for Little Brothers. Her name is Mary. Sherry's husband, Tom, is now retired and shares their visits. Mary is 95 years old and she, too, has macular degeneration. She can only see shadows. Mary lives alone in her own home and loves to go out. Sherry reflects, "A new old friend, new stories, new lessons, new reasons to be grateful."

GRATITUDE PRACTICE

Reframe your thoughts on "giving." When we think of giving, we often think of donating money to a cause. But we can give numerous other gifts, such as our time, our presence, and our caring. Consider where you can give the gift of yourself. Then think about the times you have volunteered your time and talent, and give thanks for the gift you received.

A DYNAMO WHO HELPS WOMEN FIND
THEIR WAY BACK TO THEMSELVES

Life is full of beauty. Notice it. Notice the bumble-bee, the small child, and the smiling faces. Smell the rain, and feel the wind. Live your life to the fullest potential, and fight for your dreams.

—Ashley Smith

With its prime location on the Upper East Side of Manhattan, LeMetric is the kind of hair salon where you would expect to find ladies sipping Pinot Grigio and chatting with other clients, as top-tier stylists create bouncy, layered cuts and demonstrate the mastery of blow-outs to die for. Well, it kind of is, except there are no blow dryers, and the ladies are discussing their thinning hair woes as their compassionate listener and hair caregiver, Elline Surianello, offers them green tea, gratitude, and hope.

Elline is in the business of customized care. Like so many of her customers, the 53-year-old has been living with thinning hair loss since she was in grade school. At age nine, when other girls were trying to tame their thick locks for the Marcia Brady long straight hair look, Suri-anello was diagnosed with androgenic alopecia, one of the leading causes of hair loss in females.

But instead of bemoaning her fate, Elline turned it on its ear—literally—and says she decided to be "grateful for the opportunity it gave me to help others."

After decades of finding no suitable, safe, and all-natural alternatives for her own rapid hair loss, she took it upon herself to stand up for the estimated 50 million women in the U.S. and Canada who suffer from some form of hair thinning or hair loss, and she created a viable hair loss solution. This has been the driving force behind LeMetric Inc., and it continues to be her main focus. Hair replacement pieces, along with several other beauty treatments, are offered here. And every month there are classes on hair replacement techniques and lifestyle issues.

Today, the feisty, outspoken Elline runs five affiliate salons outside her New York headquarters, in Philadelphia, Chicago, Phoenix, Toronto, and Calgary.

"Let me just start by saying that if I didn't love what I do, then there is *no* way I could do what I do," says Elline. "I help women to find solutions that satisfy their lifestyle needs."

She enthuses, "Every day is different, because every

client is different, and thus every problem or triumph is different. My clients really depend on me for more than just my tangible product. I become a confidante. It can be really difficult and very emotional, with lots of ups and downs, and I work constantly, so most people don't envy what I do. But I love it, am passionate about it, and have the joy of loving my career."

Elline says that because she has been through the struggle with hair loss herself, none of it overwhelms her at this point. "I take what my women are going through very personally. I know that I shouldn't, but I do. This is a very personal business for me; it's not just about the hair."

She says that what she likes most about what she does is helping other women feel confident in their looks. "No one assumes that working with hair is going to be life-changing, but that's exactly what it is," says Elline. "The hair is just the catalyst, and by giving women a voluptuous head of hair again, you give them their confidence, their joy, and their life back. Not everybody is prepared to do this kind of work. A lot of people have tried, but this is not your typical salon; emotions run high. It takes someone who has been through it, like me, for such a long period of time, to get to a place where you can understand all the different faces of hair loss."

She started her business at 28. Today, she is 53.

Every moment, she says, is a cause for "Thank you."

"If I had to define what I like most, I would say it's that

moment," she says. "It's that moment, after the client has gone through all of the preliminary phases, and now she is finally wearing hair for the first time. She looks in the mirror, and I see a flip in the way she holds her posture, the way she holds her head, and then the tears well up—and she tells me, this is the first time in her adult life that she has been able to look in the mirror and feel beautiful. That moment is what it's all about. It still gets me every time."

She says she is grateful for every woman who makes the choice to do something special for herself, and finds every woman who walks through her door "moving and inspirational in her own way." A lot of my clients are mothers, and as mothers, most women don't take the time out or put the money into themselves. They'll occupy themselves with their children and their schedules before they examine their own happiness and well-being. The thing is, many women don't realize that feeling good about yourself is part of being a good mother/partner/sister/friend/human."

Her work is transformative, she says, tapping into the heart and soul of women's lives. "I've had many women who come in here very bruised and battered. Either in the emotional or physical sense. I have a couple of clients who allowed themselves to be in abusive relationships for years, because they didn't believe they deserved more or that they had the strength to get out and do better. It was reclaiming their appearance, their femininity, and their womanly strength here that eventually allowed them to get out. Once they fix their insecurity, they're able to get themselves out. It's a complete transformation, really. And not just on the outside."

Elline offers this advice to women who want to empower themselves and live every day as a thank-you: "Remember this: We are always more powerful than we think we are." She adds, "If we could just give ourselves credit for living the life that we live, then we wouldn't second-guess ourselves. Once you've been over enough hurdles, you know you can deal with it. You have done it before, so you should be able to deal with it and move on."

What Elline has come to know best is the transformative power of living life as a thank-you. Instead of bemoaning our fates, she says we need to embrace them.

"The women come in with their head down, feeling a bit ashamed and unsure," she says. "When the women leave, they are full of confidence—their body language does a complete change. And at LeMetric, we're really just a community. The regular clients get to know each other. They relate in their struggles, and so the women are walking around with their hair off, being themselves, laughing, crying, whatever—and it encourages the new and potential clients that there is a way to move past this. Everyone here is grateful.

"At the beginning of the day, and at the end of the day, you have yourself, and that is the one sure thing in life," says Elline. "Along the way, you deal with a lot of inter-ference; a lot of people are going to try to sway you in different directions, and it may or may not be what you really want to do. The only way to get stronger is to go through enough life experiences, and really learn from them. Eventually, you learn how to move through the diffi-cult times smarter, faster, and more efficiently."

CULTIVATE GRATITUDE, AND BETTER HEALTH, THROUGH SERVICE TO OTHERS

A report that draws from the results of more than 30 studies on the topic of the health benefits of volunteering found that that people who volunteer have lower mortality rates, higher functional ability, and lower rates of depression.

Two of the studies indicate that there is a threshold of about 100 hours per year of volunteer activity, or about two hours per week, required to achieve a health benefit.

According to Stephen Post, director of the Institute for Research on Unlimited Love, a Case Western Reserve University research group that focuses on the scientific study of altruism, compassion, and service, you don't have to do anything dramatic. "It starts with a shift from thinking *I am the center of the world* to a willingness to act toward others in helpful ways," Post says.

Visit www.serve.gov or www.volunteermatch.org to search for volunteer opportunities by ZIP code.

THE PIANO TEACHER:
MAKING GRATEFUL MUSIC

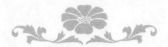

The dream begins with a teacher who believes in you, who tugs and pushes and leads you to the next plateau, sometimes poking you with a sharp stick called "truth."

—Dan Rather

Sometimes, it is our earliest mentors who taught us the lessons on new beginnings we need to learn time and again in life.

We are forever grateful for the gifts they gave us— exploring the unknown, challenging ourselves, and the confidence to go after our dreams.

When Robin Meloy Goldsby thinks about gratitude, she thinks about William Chrystal. He was her piano teacher.

She's four decades and a continent away from the time

and place of her first piano lesson, but she remembers certain details: the endless stone staircase that led to his home in the Mt. Lebanon section of Pittsburgh, the smell of his hair tonic, the way his glasses always seemed a little foggy.

By the time William Chrystal graduated from the Peabody School of Music in Baltimore—with the coveted Artist Diploma—he had earned a reputation as a perfectionist who set impossibly high standards for himself and the musicians who played with him. And his students.

"We were not excluded from his demands, his commands, his quest for perfection, his focus, drive, and absolute insistence that we *get it right*," Robin remembers. "I hardly ever got it right. I've never exhibited perfectionist traits. Ask my mother, or my husband, or anyone who has eaten one of my meals. But back then, Mr. Chrystal penetrated my nine-year-old disorganized brain and somehow convinced me that a serious study of music had nothing in common with my free-spirit approach to everything else.

" 'Music is peculiar,' he used to say. 'It takes fifteen years of hard work to find out whether or not you can play.' " All these years later, Robin understands what he meant by that puzzling statement.

The precision he required nearly drove her crazy. Often, it seemed that no amount of practice would suffice. Sometimes, she wanted to quit. "He could be nasty at lessons," Robin recalls. "Daggers would dart from behind those misty glasses of his, and he would snap at me whenever I stumbled over a phrase, or worse yet, forgot the fingering pattern he had already circled in red pencil."

Mr. Chrystal was relentless with his criticism. There were times Robin hated him. But she also admired him. Whenever she could, she would go to hear Mr. Chrystal play concerts.

He played with the Pittsburgh Symphony under the direction of William Steinberg. He was on the faculties of Carnegie Mellon University and Chatham College. He played with the Pittsburgh Ballet, the Civic Light Opera, and was a guest soloist with other symphony orchestras. And he was Robin's teacher. Robin attributes everything she's accomplished in life to him.

After leaving Pittsburgh and moving to New York, Robin built a successful career for herself as a pianist, composer, and acclaimed author, but feels that she never lived up to Mr. Chrystal's impossibly high standards.

"Bill taught his students to tame life's chaos by conquering the tricky musical passages he assigned to us," she recalls. "In our playing, he heard the sound of hope—not the smooth-edged hope of easy optimism, but hard-earned hope, the kind that comes from determination. Bill Chrystal taught me that music gives back whatever I put into it." She adds, "Music is an art that cannot be mastered, but joy—along with a healthy dose of frustration—awaits anyone who is willing to try. Four decades

154

after that first jittery lesson, I'm still reaping the benefits of his wisdom."

He's gone now, but she always hears his voice whenever she plays. "Most of the time, I still don't *get it right*, but when I do, I have him to thank," she says. "And the fact that I keep on trying, I have him to thank for that, too. Sometimes, not often enough, I catch myself playing a passage the way he would have played it, clear and perfect and full of life, and it takes my breath away. Wow, I think. Did I just do that? I wait for the nod of approval that I never got in his studio, and realize that the only nod I'll ever get will come from myself. What a beautiful gift he gave me."

GRATITUDE PRACTICE

Take some time to thank a teacher today. If your child is in school, you can write a letter to the teacher. Tell her what you appreciate about her and how your child appreciates her. Send a "report card" to the principal expressing what a great job this teacher is doing. Or honor a school by adopting a classroom and purchasing supplies, or buying books for the library. Go to www.teacherscount.org for more ideas.

CHAPTER SEVEN
FINDING GRACE AND WISDOM IN GOODBYES

Life intends Life. There is no death that is not another life beginning. There is no end that does not start anew. In every loss, in every grief, there is the hand of comfort, the hand of faith, waiting to move forward into new ways.

—Julia Cameron

One of the realities of living is that as part of humanity, we all will face heavy hits, bumps in the road that are the hard realities of life.

The truth is, life is not always fair. But in the midst of suffering and pain, we have a choice; we can affirm life and the extraordinary power of grace of which humans are capable. Or we can give in to our sadness and anger, and give up. In these stories, we find inspiration and hope—unexpected blessings—to hold us in compassion and love when we say goodbye.

In times of adversity, we are reminded how important

it is to accept that help is there for us—all we need to do is ask for it. It is then that we will find guidance, wisdom, and clarity, and know that our prayers are received and that we can be thankful that all will be well.

The challenge for us is this: how do we find the unexpected blessings in times of adversity? How do we re-vision goodbyes and loss as a doorway, an entrance to the new?

THE GOODBYE GIRL:
MY FATHER'S HOMECOMING

A grown-up daughter reflects on bringing her father home for his final days.

> *Gratitude is our most direct line to God and the angels. If we take the time, no matter how crazy and troubled we feel, we can find something to be thankful for. The more we seek gratitude, the more reason the angels will give us for gratitude and joy to exist in our lives.*
>
> —Terry Lynn Taylor

MARY BETH'S STORY

On this fall evening, I think of the moments when I *didn't* make that split-second decision to be present for someone in need.

And I thank God that I have learned to move when the moment says, "Go, now" and to try to be present when someone I love needs me.

So, this night, when my house looks as if a cyclone swooped through it, when I keep dishing out apologies to my kids and promises that life will be normal again soon (I will cook again, I will shop again, and I will clean the house again ... soon), there is one triumphant moment in our universe.

My dad is going home again. After five weeks fighting for his life in the ICU, my dad is lying on a rented hospital bed in the living room of the home he shares with my mother. He is smiling—and in hospice.

I've learned that early is better than late. I've learned that getting to the hospital fast and early is significant.

Today, I arrived in the early morning to find my dad sleeping.

He woke up. He squeezed my hand and said he had a list of things he needed me to do.

He wants me and my sister and brother to buy a birthday gift for my mom (her birthday is Halloween).

He reminded me to get him an absentee ballot so he could vote for Obama, his first Democratic vote in his 60 years as a voter.

We reviewed a list of 10 top picks of books he still wants to read, and I promised to get them in the days ahead.

And he asked me a style question: "Mary," he said, "I was watching Urlacher"—Brian Urlacher, the Chicago Bears player—"last night. Do you think I should shave off the sides so I am totally bald for this?" And he smiled.

And then he whipped off his covers and kind of moved his legs. I asked what he was doing. He said, "I am getting my clothes and going home."

He hasn't walked in 30 days. But despite it all, he has hope that he can. I told him the ambulance guys would make it easier for him now, and then he asked if he could walk when he got home.

All the people we have come to love at Hinsdale Hospital came to his room to say goodbye. We hugged and cried.

And said goodbye. Some, like the guy with the tattoos who wheeled him down for his tests, came to his room to say, "Hey, buddy, we are praying for you. We love you."

My dad just smiled his way out of there, so happy he was going home. I have learned a new talent today—how to laugh and smile and be extraordinarily happy for someone, and at the same time to have your heart ripped in two.

GRATITUDE PRACTICE

Create a prayer of farewell for a person in your life who is leaving, and a thank-you for what they have meant in your life. With each thank-you, acknowledge a gift that this person has given you. Example: Thank you, Dad, for being such a good listener. Thank you, Dad, for giving me the gift of loving to read. Then say, "We know that God goes with you."

GRATITUDE TURNS PAINFUL
MEMORIES INTO PRECIOUS GIFTS

Gratitude is the memory of the heart.

—Jean-Baptiste Massieu

Gratitude comes naturally to some people. They see the glass as half full. But most of us have to cultivate that approach to life. We live in a culture where complaining is an art form and lack of appreciation a bad habit.

Cari Stein, of Baltimore, believes she falls into the latter group, but her desire to nurture an "attitude of gratitude" is sincere and honest. She has experienced how gratitude not only changes her outlook and mood—it truly changes circumstances. What seems at the time a horrible stroke of bad luck can became an event for which we are eternally grateful.

* * *

Cari Stein was 26 at the time and had just moved to Baltimore to take on a new challenge. She had been hired for her dream job—as a producer for a network television station. Life was good.

"I remember the day, shortly after I started the job," Cari recalls. "I felt sick to my stomach. I had to go lie down in the green room and rest after the script was ready and we were about to go on air."

She ignored the symptoms because she couldn't afford to take time off work. And, she says, "I was really enjoying myself. But it got so bad I finally went to a doctor and found out I had a serious infection and needed to be hospitalized." Being new in town and alone, Cari decided to return home to a hospital in Brooklyn, New York.

"I spent the following week in a hospital, with my mother and father by my side," Cari remembers. "We played board games, cards, and talked about life. Afterward, during my recuperation, we shopped, relaxed at the local pool, and enjoyed each other's company. And once I was comfortable eating again, my father brought delicious corned beef sandwiches from my family's delicatessen. It turned out to be a special time in my life."

But what made it even more significant and poignant than she ever could have imagined is that a few months later her mother died of a heart attack. Had Cari not been ill, she would have missed out on all those special moments she shared with her parents. She understood that she had been given the gift of time with her mom, her best friend. What had appeared to be adversity became a blessing.

As it happened, Cari was not in Brooklyn the night her mother died; she had returned to Baltimore to go back to work. At 2:00 A.M. she received a call from her sister-in-law. Her mother, only 54 at the time, had died as she was getting ready for bed.

"It was a crushing blow and probably the most defining moment of my life." Cari says.

Today, 25 years later, thinking about that night still brings tears to her eyes. "But thinking about those weeks the summer before my mother died makes me smile," she says. "It turns out that my infection was no accident or coincidence, it was a gift—a chance to spend uninterrupted time with my mother, to enjoy ourselves and bask in our love for each other. For that I will be forever grateful."

GRATITUDE PRACTICE

Try the Japanese gratitude practice called Naikan, *which means "looking inside." Practitioners claim that it helps people understand themselves and their relationships, and put things into better perspective. Cari Stein was able to find the gift in her situation. The practice involves asking yourself these three questions:*

What have I received from this person?
What have I given to this person?
What troubles and difficulties have I caused to this person?

RECONCILING SADNESS
AND LOSS WITH GRATITUDE

Find the good—and praise it.

—Alex Haley

We all struggle with the act of letting go—whether it's physically letting go of material goods, emotionally detaching from people who have hurt us, losing a job, or saying goodbye and moving on when someone we love has died. Sometimes gratitude is less about striving than it is about surrendering.

In this story, Ruth Perryman discovers that during a time of great suffering, when she lost her son and it seemed her well of hope had run dry, she discovered gratitude. She learned to say thank you for the wake-up call after her tragic loss. It brought her to appreciate the incredible gift of her family and her seven other children.

Difficult though it can be to understand, it is gratitude that gets us through stressful times and painful endings. Ruth learned to say thank you, even when it felt forced. Being grateful helps us stop trying to control what will happen and unlocks positive energy in our lives. Sadness and loss can become blessings and bring unexpected gifts.

Ruth Perryman was a busy professional woman with eight children. The Roseville, California, mother had carved out a life juggling family and work, rising through the ranks of two nonprofits to become chief financial officer.

The long hours advanced her career. They were not without sacrifice, leaving little time for her husband, Randy, and eight children. But the trade-offs somehow made it seem worth it—plenty of money in the bank, a nice home, nice cars (even an RV and a Honda Gold Wing motorcycle), and the kids had everything they could want.

Unfortunately, this American Dream came crashing down when their 21-year old son, Brian, accidentally over-dosed on an over-the-counter pain-killer taken to treat his chronic rheumatoid arthritis, and died.

"The shock caused us to reevaluate the way we were living our lives," Ruth recalls. "We found ourselves anxious when we were at work, and our youngest children (aged eight and nine at the time) started experiencing problems at school because they couldn't shake the feeling we might not come home that night."

The family started making changes gradually—first by working out a deal with Ruth's employer to allow her to work from home so she could homeschool the kids for the last few months of the school year.

The following September, they enrolled their children in a charter school and tried to go back to their former lives. Even though Ruth worked fewer hours in the office, it just wasn't enough. She knew she needed to make family a greater priority. The family made a collective decision to overhaul their lifestyle—downsize their expenses—and move back to Ruth's hometown, Sacramento, where most of her extended family lived, and she began to homeschool her children full-time.

"It wasn't easy," Ruth remembers. "My husband was lucky enough to find a telecommuting position with his employer, but I had to resign from my position because my employer really needed someone in the office. I tried to find another job closer to our new home, but the economy was already starting to slide so I decided to focus on my QuickBooks consulting practice, which I'd started back in 1996. There were moments when we were terrified about our decision: would we be able to survive on just my husband's salary, and did we damage our kids by moving away from the only home they'd ever known?"

It's now been nearly two years since their son Brian

died. Ruth says that the family misses him every day, but they are grateful for the gift he gave them.

"My business is thriving—I even continue doing remote consulting for my former employer," says Ruth. "In fact, I now make much more money than I ever did as an employee. And more importantly, I now spend 24 hours a day, 7 days a week with my husband and children. This might drive some people crazy, but I've never seen our kids happier or more secure."

The loss of her son's life helped Ruth and her family see the gift of grace in every moment, and she accepts all this with great gratitude.

"I guess you can say this is our son's last gift to us. He opened our eyes to what was really important—before it was too late."

GRATITUDE PRACTICE
Start your day with this intention:

> *Today, I will be grateful. I will start the process of turning today's pain into tomorrow's joy.*
> —*from* The Language of Letting Go, *by Melody Beattie*

GRATITUDE AS A SECOND CHANCE

Dorothea Hover-Kramer, a psychotherapist and author of six books, including *Second Chance at Your Dream: Engaging Your Body's Energy Resources for Optimal Aging, Creativity and Health,* believes in the transformative power of gratitude.

She says: "Being thankful changes our energy from demanding to appreciation. Instead of increasing our expectations of how things should be, we can move toward recognizing what is. I like learning from my pets—every caring gesture or morsel of food is appreciated. It's important to stay in touch with the reality of how much we've been given!"

MY GRANDMOTHER'S HUGS

In giving thanks for the past, we move forward.

> *I awoke this morning with devout thanksgiving for my friends, the old and the new.*
> —Ralph Waldo Emerson

There is no denying the grandma factor. Though many of us long ago said goodbye to these auxiliary parents in our lives, specific little moments—the smell of a favorite food, a Christmas tree ornament, a photo—transport us back over the years and we find ourselves awash in gratitude for what our grandparents meant to us.

A hugging touch of care, an act of love, helps us to focus not on the absence of those we loved, but rather on our sincere gratitude and heartfelt feelings for the role they played in our lives.

Here, Michele Kirk, of San Francisco, reminds us to be grateful for those in our lives who are past and present.

We all carry with us memories that we can tap into when we want to get in touch with thanksgiving. When we're not having a good day, all it takes is an inward look at our most valued relationships—past and present—to feel thankful and uplifted.

Michele Kirk is a single woman in her mid-thirties, a psychotherapist in private practice who is now helping families of divorce transition smoothly through change. She is grateful for the people who have loved her, for those who have supported her on her journey and been a guiding force in her life. Although, like so many of us, she has experienced loss, she has not lost the connections made in her heart, and she cherishes the memories of people like her big Gramma: Grams, Gertie, G-Love.

"She passed away this past summer, and I miss her so," Michele says. "I miss her big Gramma hugs that were part soft, cushy landing, and part death grip. I miss the big family gatherings she organized, where she was determined to make everyone's favorite dish. I miss her open-door policy and the security of knowing that she was always available to me.

"But when things are rough, I know that I still have her with me. I cannot erase the years of love and support that she has given me and the guidance she provided that has shaped the woman I am today. These gifts are a comfort to me now, especially during challenging times."

Michele says she has internalized her grandma's love and support, especially her encouraging messages: "Keep trying," "We know you can do it," "We're so proud of you," and the most important by far, "Remember that Gramma and Grampa love you very much."

Michele's grandma was one of her biggest fans, and a constant positive force in her life; she helped buffer Michele through some very difficult times, including her parents' divorce when she was seven.

"It was my gramma who took me under her loving wing," she recalls. "This often involved long phone calls when I was mad at my parents, sad about their separation, or when I was missing my father. My gramma was always reachable, and I could call her anytime to talk.

"As a child in the seventies, both of my parents worked, which left me home alone before and after school. In the mornings I would get ready for school, and then call my gramma, who would talk with me until it was time to leave for school, and then remind me to take my lunch and jacket, and lock the door.

"When I'd call after a bad day—a speeding ticket, a bad grade, a breakup—she'd remind me, 'Tomorrow is a new day, and Gramma and Grampa love you very much.'

"And when I'd call her, bored and restless, she would stay on the phone with me for hours, never saying that she had to go. Sometimes she would make up games for us to play, she at her house and I at mine, and then we would talk again in a few hours to see who won. I imagine that this was a way for her to buy some time off the phone, but she never said that. She was always there for me, whatever I needed, whenever I needed it. We would always end our calls with 'love ya,' and if one of us forgot, the other would call back just to say it."

After her grandmother died, there was an empty space where she had been, Michele remembers. She took a couple of things to keep her grandma's memory alive: a Danish cookbook, a Christmas tree ornament, and an old dress from the 1950s that she found in her attic.

"I recently tried on that dress, and it fit perfectly," says Michele. "In that act, I could feel my grandmother right there with me. I felt her big Gramma hug. I heard her praises and encouragement.

"My heart swelled with love and gratitude for her place in my life. I knew that she was still available to me, and that I could access her at any moment through simple means like looking at her photo, listening to her favorite song, or trying on her dress from days gone by.

"It is moments like this that inspire me, and propel me forward, even in hard times, because that's what we do," Michele says. "We keep moving forward."

GRATITUDE PRACTICE
The Christian writer G. K. Chesterton had the right idea when he said we need to get in the habit of "taking things

with gratitude and not taking things for granted." Write a letter to your relatives acknowledging the special role a relative who is now gone has played in your family circle. Ask them to say a prayer of thanksgiving for this person and the legacy he or she has left for all of you.

CHAPTER EIGHT

INSPIRATION AND PERSPIRATION:
ALL PARTS GRATITUDE

If you can imagine it, you can achieve it; if you can dream it, you can become it.

—William Arthur Ward

Daring deeds and great accomplishments often start with a lightbulb moment—a bright idea that takes hold and illuminates our path.

Whether we start on our journey full of appreciation, or embark on one to seek inspiration and fulfillment, gratitude is the driving force that brings us closer to our goals.

AFTER A RACE AROUND THE WORLD, A MOM OPENS UP TO GRATITUDE AND PAYS IT FORWARD

The greatest part of our happiness depends on our dispositions, not our circumstances.

—Martha Washington

What would go through your mind after being deposited in the Mongolian desert, blindfolded, after a 22-hour flight, with two strangers, a 50-pound backpack filled with camping gear, camera equipment, McDonald's gift certificates, a hundred dollars, and marching orders to make your way back to New York City?

In this story, Tami Becker, of Piedmont, California, tells us how her thoughts turned to gratitude as she found her way back to her loving family.

Tami Becker counts her blessings every day. A mother of four from Piedmont, California, and an active volunteer who runs a foundation for cystic fibrosis, Tami has held the hands of friends and family as they battled illness and loss, yet she is filled with gratitude every day for her health, and her husband and family.

In 2001, Tami was at home raising four children. She relished the work and the rewards, but as she says, "When friends began reentering the workplace, I made the decision to stay home, but I needed a change. I needed to feel appreciated, and I needed to appreciate. I needed to miss my family, and they needed to miss me, so I embarked on the ultimate adventure." She landed herself a role as a contestant on a short-lived reality TV show on NBC called *Lost*. Her mission was to race against two other teams of two back to the Statue of Liberty in New York.

After the plane landed in a completely unknown destination, Tami recounts, she was paired with a woman named Celeste and a videographer.

"We could have been on the dark side of the moon. The landscape was completely barren, and we were surrounded by hills. As we made our way out of the desert, it became clear that many of the things in our packs were useless."

They soon learned that all they really needed was their own resourcefulness and the ability to ask for, and accept, acts of kindness from strangers.

"Our first kindness was a Mongolian man whose family lived in a yurt; he took care of us for the night and offered us lodging. We set up our tent in the middle of his herd of goats, and filtered his precious water into our Nalgene bottles. He then strapped all of our gear to his one motorcycle and drove it thirty miles to the nearest town, assuring us with hand signals, since we had no other common language between us, that he would meet us there when we arrived.

"We had no idea if we would ever see our belongings again, but we had faith, and as we hiked our way in the midday sun across the Mongolian desert on foot, faith kept us moving. He met us along a stretch of the road leading into a small settlement and helped us to get a ride to the next town, where we pleaded our way into a tiny room with no hot water. We had to squat at a faucet on the floor to rinse off the sweat and desert dust, but we were thrilled for the respite from the desert."

Other moments of gratitude abounded. She especially remembers the day they witnessed a van identical to theirs turned over, with the carnage of bodies surrounding it.

"We had arrived during a special Mongolian holiday," Tami recalls. "There were vans hauling people and supplies across the desert on treacherous uneven routes. There were no markers to indicate rocks or holes, and the contents of our van were tossed about like a shaker of dice. It could just as easily been us; it was just a matter of chance which van wasn't going to reach its destination safely. That night we ran into another team, and we were all so happy to have survived that we embraced one another, pooled our resources, and split a room at an actual hotel."

The villages and people became poorer and poorer, yet the people continued to embrace Tami and her partner.

Today, she continues to be grateful for the Russian reporter who gave up her savings to provide Tami and her team the money for a boat to transport them to their next destination. Mormon American boys helped out by translating for them for a couple of days. Two women gave them a place to stay, and even helped to celebrate Celeste's birthday. A young man spent the equivalent of almost a week's salary to buy Tami and Celeste lunch. The list goes on.

"My self-absorbed quest for adventure quickly became a reality check on the beauty and ills of the human spirit," recalls Tami. "As we lived day to day on the kindness of strangers, I was reminded of how many people there are who have nothing in this world."

As for the young man who bought them lunch? That was the breaking point for Tami. She had no idea how much it truly cost him, and when someone translated it for her, she broke down and cried.

"Here I was in his country, trying to get back to one of the wealthiest countries in the world, to win a prize of more money and a car that I didn't even need, while one young man had to work so hard to have enough money to buy me lunch. Something was wrong, so terribly wrong with this picture, and so I cried. I cried so hard that I could hardly breathe, and of course the camera guy followed me, thrilled to have footage of the drama, and NBC played it again and again in the ads for the show. But I was not crying because I was scared or alone or because I missed my family. I was crying because I was ashamed and embarrassed. How could I win more of anything when people who had nothing were giving me everything they could?"

Today, Tami reflects on that experience.

"I'm overwhelmed by the feeling of gratitude for the kindness of others, and the realization that first and foremost you have to want what you have," she says. "I came in second the day that I touched ground at the Statue of Liberty, but I got the biggest prize that anyone could have hoped for. It was gratitude."

These days, she practices gratitude by showing the good grace and kindness that others showed her on her journey through the desert. She thinks of her reality TV experience as a metaphorical journey to find strength in her choices and solidify the things that she appreciates in her life. The experience has helped to transform her and given her the grace to be thankful for every moment of every day. Mostly, it has taught her to give back from that place of gratitude.

She says, "When I am out and about, I look at the homeless and the panhandlers differently now. I have felt that hunger, and hope. So I wish them a good day, and hand them some help. I often fold singles individually and slip them in my back pocket for easy access. I always bring water out to the gal in front of my local grocery store.

"Last week, when it was particularly cold, I told the guy at the coffee shop to make it two and I handed one to the lady with the 'Save the Children' collection tin out front. We chatted for a moment, and I was rewarded with a perfect smile. In the end, I guess it is rather selfish of me, buying smiles for only a buck, a cup of tea, or by simply acknowledging someone, but I figure it is a two-way street, and we all need to feel a bit of gratitude."

GRATITUDE PRACTICE
If you travel outside the U.S. to a Third World country, take the time to get out of the resort, off the tourist track, and experience the local culture. Put away your credit card, buy from the locals, talk to the indigenous people, and take note of what makes them happy.

ACHIEVING THE AMERICAN DREAM

> Not knowing when the dawn will come, I open
> every door.
>
> —Emily Dickinson

José Ayllon, a native of Toluca, México, grew up the second
to youngest of 10 children. To support his children, José's
dad went to the United States to work and send money
back. At 14, José moved six hours away to live with an
elder sibling in Guanajuato. He was seeking independence
and tried to juggle high school and working full-time. It
didn't work, and José ended up dropping out of school.

Two years later, his father phoned asking his son to move
to the United States. So at 16, José and two of his older
sisters joined their father in Pennsylvania.

"The plan was to work together for a few months and save some money so my mom and little brother could come here as well so we could all live together," says José. "When I was making my decision about coming to the U.S., I thought about everything except the language barrier. Not knowing the language made things extremely difficult for me. I could not find a job, because most of the jobs I applied for required some level of English."

His father kept urging José to return to school. But José had other plans, and instead went to work at a mushroom farm, working every day from 4:00 A.M. to 5:00 P.M.

His dad persisted on the education campaign front. "My dad did not seem very happy with my decision and kept encouraging me to go to school," José says.

Sadly, about four months after José and his sisters moved in with their father, their dad was critically injured in a car accident and died two weeks later.

"My life lost direction when that happened," José says. "I had no idea where to start and how to start. We ended up going back to Mexico to bury my dad. Once the family gathered together, we decided to come back to the U.S. with my mom, my younger brother, two of my older brothers and their families, and two of my sisters."

Back in the U.S., José heeded his father's advice and started high school as a sophomore.

"I knew that learning the language was going to be one of the biggest challenges. I was very lucky to have excellent teachers of English as a second language. They were always encouraging me to perform to the best of my ability. Thanks to their help and with a lot of hard work, within a year I had learned the language."

José's teachers encouraged him to become part of a leadership group representing his high school. José and a team of four students attended a conference in Pennsylvania, with the challenge to create a plan for their community. The group decided to focus on improving culture awareness. Despite his struggle with the English language, José came up with the project's title: P.E.A.C.E. UNION, which stands for "people enthusiastic about cultural equality."

The project focused on creating language exchange classes, which the team called "Intercambio classes."

The group held the classes once a week after school for the large Spanish-speaking population. "Our project was a huge success," José enthuses. "Within a few months we decided to extend the program to our community in general. Once again, in our community it proved to be a success as well and is still in place today. This wonderful project won us first place statewide. That program really made a difference in my life. I suddenly realized that when you really want something and you work to achieve it, anything is possible."

José got into the giving-back aspect of the project and found himself finding numerous ways to become involved in his community. He worked with the Migrant Education Program as a summer teacher's assistant, helping students from Mexico who have just arrived in the United States.

"I felt proud to be able to help students that were in the same position I once was in," he says. He also worked at the Garage Youth Center as a tutor and mentor for high school students. "However, as graduation got closer and closer, I was not sure if I was going to be able to pursue my dream to attend Marywood University. My financial situation was not the best. I had to apply for a lot of different scholarships in order to be able to afford to attend."

Today, he is a senior at Marywood and is determined to graduate and pursue a career that makes a difference in others' lives. He knows his dad would be smiling at his myriad activities—the Dean's List every semester, the Diversity United International Club, the World Language Club, the ACT 101 program; the Chi Alpha Epsilon honor society, tutoring, and serving as master of ceremonies for a leadership breakfast.

"I am very proud of everything I have achieved and I am very thankful for all the help I have received throughout all this time," says José. "I now look back and I see my younger brother, nephews, and nieces extremely motivated about pursing a higher education. One of my nephews is now a junior at Indiana University of Pennsylvania; my niece is a sophomore at Villanova; and my younger brother is a freshman at Penn State University. The rest of my nephews and nieces are mostly in high school and they, as well, are very interested about pursuing a college career. I feel very proud to see that, thanks to the things I have been able to accomplish, they have seen that it is possible to achieve a goal, when you work for it to make it come true.

"I am very proud to know that I am an inspiration to my family members, just as my parents and the rest of my family have been my inspiration to succeed," he adds.

What's next? José is considering becoming a lawyer or studying for an MBA. Money continues to be a challenge, but he is approaching this with a spirit of gratitude for what will be his next dream come true.

These days he is very grateful to the William G. McGowan scholarship fund, which is paying for one year of José's business school education. The funds are requested by the university and the money granted to that college, which must have an accredited business school. The business school faculty judges the essays and chooses the student to receive the scholarship based on their essays and financial need. The funds are used by the university for the winning student, either for their senior year as a business major or for a year in a business master's program.

José was selected because his presentation to the business faculty was the most impressive and promising.

"I applied for this scholarship and a few months later I received a letter congratulating me for winning," he says. "That moment and that call changed my life and my future completely. This academic year I have been able to fully focus on my studies without having to constantly be worried about my financial situation. Today I still do not have enough words to thank everyone involved in this wonderful fund, for changing my life and my future the way they did. All I can say is that it has been an honor to be the recipient of such a prestigious award."

THE LUCK OF THE IRISH: SHINING THE POWER OF GRATITUDE INTO A LIFE-GIVING FORCE

Silent gratitude isn't much use to anyone.

—G.B. Stern

It started as a casual conversation between friends, a group of guys gathered at a pub in New York City, who felt they were pretty lucky and wanted to help those who weren't. They felt they needed to give thanks for what they had by helping others.

They decided to help kids with cancer. The St. Baldrick's Foundation was founded in 1999, when the trio shaved off their heads and asked for pledges from their circle of friends. (The title is a takeoff on the name of the popular Irish saint, St. Patrick.)

In 10 years, the Foundation has exploded into the

world's biggest volunteer-driven fundraising program for childhood cancer. Events are held across the globe, typically in March each year around St. Patrick's Day, and thousands of folks volunteer to organize the community parties. Professional hair stylists or friends and families with shavers shave the heads of volunteers to raise funds for kids with cancer. During the last decade, St. Baldrick's events (www.StBaldricks.org) have taken place in 18 countries and 48 states, raising over $50 million and shaving more than 72,000 heads.

In 1999, Tim Kenny challenged his friends John Bender and Enda McDonnell to find a way to give back to society. These three reinsurance executives turned their industry's St. Patrick's Day party into a benefit for kids with cancer. What could they do to really turn the heads—and the wallets—of their colleagues?

John suggested shaving Enda's head, since kids typically lose their hair during cancer treatment. "People will gladly pay to see you bald, Enda!" Never one to miss an opportunity, Enda replied, "I will if you will," and St. Baldrick's was born.

The three planned to raise "$17,000 on the 17th," recruiting 17 colleagues to raise $1,000 each to be shorn. Instead, the first St. Baldrick's event, held on March 17, 2000, raised over $104,000!

"We were just sitting around at a bar and we started

talking about how lucky we were in our own lives," says Tim. "We thought, hey, we should do something to show how grateful we are for what we have, and we should do something for others who are struggling."

At a St. Baldrick's event, something amazing happens, Tim says. People who normally shy away from the very thought of childhood cancer find themselves compelled to support this cause after looking into the faces of these brave children who are smiling broadly as their friends and family members proudly display their newly shorn heads.

In March 2009, Tim witnessed the pay-it-forward power of the trio's gift of gratitude in action. More than 1,000 people had packed the Hanging Gardens Banquet Hall in River Grove, Illinois, in honor of one girl—Maggie Horn. At six years old, Maggie, then in kindergarten, had been diagnosed with acute lymphocytic leukemia.

But Maggie's parents, Bill and Barb, stayed focused when they got the diagnosis, pledging, "We'll get you through this. We are a family team, and we are in this all together." And they did, through two and a half years of countless blood draws, spinal taps, and bone marrow draws, as well as chemotherapy treatments.

Three years ago, like the trio of guys who felt they were lucky and founded St. Baldrick's, the Horn family decided that they wanted to say thank you to everyone who had helped support them on their journey through Maggie's cancer.

"We felt the best way to express our gratitude would be to help other families who were facing what we did," says Barb.

What started as a gathering of a group of fireman from Bill Horn's firehouse in Franklin Park has exploded into a megafundraising event, with more than 1,000 people raising $102,000 for critically ill kids with cancer. (The Horns and their team of organizers had set a goal of $65,000, thinking it was ambitious for the tough economic times of spring 2009, but they surpassed it by $37,000.) The event has expanded to include firemen, paramedics, and police officers and their families from a handful of western suburban Chicago towns.

Today, Maggie is vivacious 13-year-old who plays catcher on a travel softball team. The Horn family—Maggie, her parents, older brother Ryan, and little sis Allie—are an unstoppable fundraising force.

At a time when it gets exhausting to hear about all the gloom and doom, the actions of Tim Kenny and the Horn family speak volumes about the power of being grateful for the blessings in life, and how, in giving from that gratitude, we can spread it to others.

The impact of three guys sitting on bar stools who stood up and took action speaks for itself: in 2008, St. Baldrick's events were hosted in 48 U.S. states in addition to Australia, Bermuda, Brazil, Canada, Hong Kong, India, Iran, Iraq, Mexico, Northern Ireland, and the

United Kingdom, and more events are signing up daily as the movement continues to spread.

In 2008, St. Baldrick's donors and volunteers made possible over $15 million in funding for childhood cancer research. This includes 47 grants, as well as funding for 30 young doctors who will be tomorrow's top researchers. In addition, tens of thousands of volunteers make St. Baldrick's happen, with the leadership of a board of directors and the support of a small staff. Volunteers organize each event, coached and equipped by the foundation.

Shavees and volunteers can participate in honor of kids who are fighting cancer or in memory of kids who have waged the fight. These children and teens give a face and a story to the cause, inspiring all to go the extra mile (or inch, in terms of hair) in raising funds and awareness.

FOOD FOR THOUGHT: CAFÉ GRATITUDE
PROVIDES SUSTENANCE FOR BODY AND SOUL

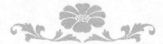

*By saying grace, we release the Divine sparks in
our food.*

—Rabbi Herschel

*Consider Terces and Matthew Engelhart the Martha
Stewarts of gratitude. When they met, the San Francisco
area couple committed to living their lives from a place of
inner guidance, no matter how crazy it seemed in the "Me
decade" of the 1980s.*

*Out of that determination to guide their future through
the practices of abundance, love, acceptance, and gratefulness, the couple found a winning recipe to serve up
gratitude—with nourishment. In 2004, they brought to
life that concept when they opened Café Gratitude in the
Mission District of San Francisco.*

Now there are seven locations (with plans for expansion), and every order on the menu is an affirmation: "I am Worthy," "I am Giving," and "I am Grateful."

When Terces and Matthew Engelhart started turning to their gut and inner voice for guidance, their first instinct was to create a transformational board game called "The Abounding River." The purpose of the game was to help people transform from a place of scarcity to a place of abundance. Introducing the board game and a book based on the same principles, the couple started leading game-based workshops across the country. That led to the idea of opening a place where people could gather and play the game.

"We wanted to create lives for ourselves where we practiced 'being abundance,' and not living out of the survival and scarcity mode," recalls Matthew. "We realized early on that abundance and gratitude go hand in hand. We wanted to focus our intention on gratefulness. And we wanted also to help others consciously practice this and to create a community that reminded us to support each other."

Café Gratitude was born and became the couple's expression of a world of plenty. The idea of gratitude spread like wildfire. Today, six years later, 230 employees are part of the Café Gratitude family, and 1,500 customers walk through the doors of the seven locations every day, ringing up sales of $21,000 daily.

"Our customers come from all walks of life," Terces says. "They come to us because they have a shared intention of making every day a day of thanksgiving. Regardless of their circumstances, whether they have cancer, or have lost their jobs, or no matter what, they want to keep their intentions on being grateful. These people here are living extraordinary lives and celebrating it."

Terces and Matthew and those who have found a home at Café Gratitude share a common belief: "When times get tough, you give more," Matthew says. In 2009, in an effort to help those hurt by the suffering economy, Café Gratitude eateries launched a program called the "I Am Grateful Bowl." Customers who can afford to eat and want to help others donate funds in a jar at the front of the restaurants. Those who can't afford a meal can come to the restaurants and say, "I Am Grateful," and they are served a free meal.

"Our food and people are a celebration of our aliveness," Terces says. At Café Gratitude eateries, diners select the finest organic ingredients to honor the earth and ourselves, as we are one and the same. They support local farmers, sustainable agriculture, and environmentally friendly products. And the food is prepared with love.

The menu's cover reads: "We invite you to step inside and enjoy being someone who chooses: loving your life, adoring yourself, accepting the world, being generous and grateful every day, and experiencing being provided for."

GRATITUDE PRACTICE

Terces offers this practice, which she calls Rewriting Your Life. Consider that you know who you are, how you react, what triggers you—you even warn other people about the ways you are. You might also be quietly waiting for people to figure out who you are, again already knowing. But what if you could create yourself newly every day? What if you could start saying things about yourself that create you as more of who you really want to be? Maybe you can. I invite you to take it on. For just one week, pick a way of being that perhaps you don't think you are and start affirming that way. Let's say, for example, I am beautiful or I am generous. Pick one that you aspire to but don't think you are quite there yet.

Now, for a whole week, really take on practicing being this way. Look yourself in the mirror first thing each morning—every time you get into the car, look into that mirror, before you go to sleep at night again, look into the mirror and repeat your affirmation. Keep it up all week long. Notice your experience as the week progresses. Let what you are saying sink in, stop resisting it, just breathe into your words. At the end of the week, ask yourself, How was that for you? What are you present to now? How do you see and experience yourself?

You can rewrite your life. Whatever story you are telling yourself and others, if it empowers you, great, keep sharing it. If it doesn't empower you, start practicing

sharing another story. Make one up that is empowering—
you made up one that wasn't, so why not make up one
that is? Go ahead, let yourself fall in love with yourself—
and with everyone else in your life, too.

WEATHER REPORT
by BJ Gallagher

"Any day I'm vertical
is a good day"
—that's what I always say.
And I give thanks
that I'm healthy.
If you ask me,
"How are you?"
I'll answer, "GREAT!"
because in saying so,
I make it so.
And I give thanks
that I can choose my attitude.
When Life gives me dark clouds and rain,
I appreciate the moisture
which brings a soft curl to my hair.
When Life gives me sunshine,
I gratefully turn my face up
to feel its warmth on my cheeks.
When Life brings fog,
I hug my sweater around me
and give thanks for the cool shroud of mystery

that makes the familiar seem different and intriguing.
When Life brings snow,
I dash outside to catch the first flakes on my tongue,
relishing the icy miracle that is a snowflake.
Life's events and experiences
are like the weather—
they come and go,
no matter what my preference.
So, what the heck?!
I might as well decide to enjoy them.
For indeed,
there IS a time for every purpose
under Heaven.
Each season brings its own unique blessings.
And I give thanks.

CHAPTER NINE
GRATITUDE IN TIMES OF TRANSITION

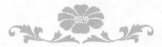

What if you gave someone a gift, and they neglect-
ed to thank you for it—would you be likely to give
them another? Life is the same way. In order to
attract more of the blessings that life has to offer,
you must truly appreciate what you already have.

—Ralph Marston

At some point in our lives, we've all been told to look for
the blessings in times of upheaval and confusion, as often
is the case when we're ending a relationship, moving to a
new job, or facing a life passage. But it is hard in transition
not to be pessimistic when the future is so uncertain, or
when we've lost something or someone we love.

Transitions can electrify the air with fearfulness. That's
because in transitions, you're taking apart the structure of
the life you know and preparing to rebuild it into something new.

Unfortunately, the more we focus on our fears and the

lack of what is existing in our lives the scarier and more depressing things get. How can we expect more in the future if we don't appreciate what we already have? We need to humble ourselves and look at what we do have to be grateful for, even if something cherished is now missing. What we are experiencing in transition is temporary and this too will pass.

When we focus on our blessings and look forward to what lies ahead with a spirit of hope, it can help us mobilize the courage and the heart to open the gates of tenderness, right in the midst of fear and uncertainty. Then we can see transition times as opportunities for tremendous growth in our lives.

Consider the words of Lee Woodruff, reflecting on the months after her husband, the reporter Bob Woodruff, was injured in Iraq: "Thankfully, there inevitably comes a period in time when you begin to move away from the eye of the hurricane. No matter what the outcome, you let out your breath and learn to operate once again outside of the crisis mode. It's the point in time when you have to put one tentative foot in front of the other and widen the distance between you and the first horrible piece of news."

In times of transition, we need to tap into the transforming power of gratefulness. Here, we see the inner shifts that happen as people find their lives moving through the unknown to what is about to unfold.

MAKING ROOM FOR THE MYSTERY: UNLOCKING THE POWER OF GRATITUDE IN ILLNESS

> *Gratitude unlocks the fullness of life. It turns what we have into enough, and more. It turns denial into acceptance, chaos into order, and confusion into clarity. It turns problems into gifts, failures into success, the unexpected into perfect timing, and mistakes into important events. Gratitude makes sense of our past, brings peace for today, and creates a vision for tomorrow."*
>
> —Melodie Beattie

In the midst of her rich and abundant life, Carol Levinson admits she experienced adventures and happiness in ways most of us would envy. In that ordinary, yet extraordinary living, Carol says she received a great deal more than she could ever hope to give.

Until illness struck, forcing her to stop in the middle of an agenda-filled life. Then she had to consciously seek how abundance was working in her life by shifting her perspective and finding gratitude in the simple rhythms of the day. Carol found that the easiest and most effective

*way of moving through tough times was to pause and find
the beauty in her garden, her pets, the love of her husband,
and the resilience and spunk of her 93-year-old mother.*

Carol Levinson projects a radiant aura that immediately
lights up a room. So it's not surprising when she tells you
she has long studied energy fields, and can levitate and
move inanimate objects.

Growing up in the small town of Clarence Center, near
Buffalo, New York, Carol always felt that everything came
easy to her. "I was a lucky kid and took my abilities for
granted," she says. "I was aware of my family members'
severe colon issues, but even after developing symptoms, it
didn't stop me from accomplishing my goals."

Carol went on to lead a life that many of us only
fantasize about: she joined the Peace Corps; sang and
danced in theater troupes; lived in a utopian community
in Mendocino, California; traveled the world working on
cruise ships; and rose to prominent positions in the fields
of nursing and teaching.

"I've led a charmed life despite suffering from ulcerative colitis," she recalls. "Until the day in 2005 when I
was diagnosed with cancer. That's when I had to turn to
other people for support. I give thanks every day for the
love of my caring husband."

She is mostly upset about the fact that she had to give
up working. "All my life I've helped others," she says.

"Now that I'm not working, I feel like I'm not doing all I can to make a difference."

After getting a master's in nursing, Carol taught at the University of Pennsylvania in Philadelphia and then transferred to San Francisco to teach at the UCSF School of Nursing. She lived in the famed Haight-Ashbury neighborhood of San Francisco and took up massage therapy and energy healing. She studied Buddhism and meditation.

Then, one day, she cast aside her tenured position and city apartment to move to Oz, a hippie commune located on a huge ranch bordered by redwood forests on the pristine Garcia River near Point Arena, in Mendocino County, California.

"After living there for three years, I became consumed with the idea of working on a cruise ship. But after many attempts and no call-backs, I gave up the idea."

Carol describes a summer solstice ceremony where she created a prayer arrow composed of found objects wound around a stick, which was then thrown into a fire. She was giving up her intention of cruising the world. But that very evening, Sitmar (now Princess Lines and Holland America) called and hired her on the spot. So Carol went from tofu and sprouts to a life of Champagne and baked Alaska. She loved her life on the seas, working as a massage therapist and nurse, but gave it up as her colitis got worse. She moved back to San Francisco and in 1992 met and married her "knight in shining armor," Ted Levinson. She was 50.

By 2005, after having tried every alternative healing treatment known, she was on a heavy course of steroids. During a week of severe flare-ups she showed up every day at Kaiser Permanente's Urgent Care Center to plead for a colonoscopy. When a raw ulcer turned out to be a cancerous tumor, it didn't surprise her. She was immediately scheduled for an emergency sigmoid resection and chemotherapy.

From January to August 2008, Carol received three separate treatments of intravenous chemotherapy to reduce the inflammation. With each successive treatment, there were serious side effects. The last treatment resulted in an unexpected, profound hypertensive reaction. Her blood pressure rose so high that her coronary arteries were impaired. A week later, Carol woke with excruciating chest pain and experienced three heart attacks in a row. To add insult to injury, chronic ulcerative colitis is frequently associated with painful autoimmune inflammatory arthritis, so she had to deal with the side effects of pain medication as well. The end result is that she can no longer work and has days when she is unable to leave the house.

Carol attributes her ability to "keep on keeping on" to gratitude. "I am so grateful that I have the spiritual tools to keep me living in each moment!" she exclaims. "I don't pretend that everything is wonderful. My husband tells me that I cry out in the night. Really, what choice does one have but to 'put your boots on' and keep going, one step at a time."

Carol is grateful for the support of her wonderful husband, her pets, her friends, her peaceful garden in bucolic Marin County, California, and her spry 93-year-old mother. She has begun to work with color, painting faces and bodies, fabric and ceramics, and she enjoys cooking. She is hopeful that in six months she will be stable enough to have surgery for the placement of an ileostomy. Carol yearns to participate in life and become more active. Remembering to feel gratitude for her blessings reduces the sadness and redirects the focus from all that she has lost.

Although she can no longer work professionally as a nurse, Carol continues to devise ways to help others, such as nurturing and holding sick children, or visiting with the elderly to sing and tell stories. Many people would be bitter if they were handed these genetic cards. Grateful people like Carol show us that a spirit of giving has its own psychic rewards. The practice of gratitude is a tool we may all depend upon to meet life's challenges with courage and grace.

GRATITUDE PRACTICE
Practice gratitude affirmations. Create your own: "I am grateful that..." or "I am grateful for..." Check out www. GratitudeKit.com for a full resource on affirmations you can use every day.

GRATEFUL FOR THE END OF A UNION AND THE BEGINNING OF THE SELF

Praise the bridge that carried you over.

—George Colman

Whoever possesses an enlightened sense of self in a time of loss will be blessed with happiness. Or at least that is the hope and defense we'd like to hang on to when we are forced by life's circumstances to begin again.

If we want to boost our stamina for starting over, we might look to the wisdom of Michele Woodward. Michele is living proof that tuning in to an attitude of gratitude during times when we want to jump into bed and hide under the covers is the best way to feel better, inside and out.

Michele shares the secret to revitalizing yourself, getting back to clarity, and calming yourself so as to begin again, with purpose, passion, and gratefulness for the opportunity. It is gratitude for all, she says, that gives us the inner compass to point us in the direction we need to go—forward.

If you had told Michele Woodward, in what she calls "those protracted prostrate sessions" when she lay on the ice-cold tile in the bathroom crying her eyes out, that someday she would feel grateful that her husband left her for a younger woman he met on the Internet, she would have told you that you were crazy.

"If you had said, 'This, too, shall pass,' I might have scratched your eyes out," recalls Michele, a mother of two from Arlington, Virginia. "If you had urged balance and sangfroid, I would have impaled you on the plumber's helper."

It was not a good time.

"I was in no mood to hear about the future," she recalls. "I had lost my future. Because my vision of the future did not include him as my husband. And how would I, dumped as 'too old' at 43, fill the big hole he was leaving in my life? I had been his wife for many years and his girlfriend before that. I had taken his name, and his life. And now he had taken all of that from me. And given it to someone else."

She adds, "I felt robbed. I felt cheated. I felt abandoned."

"Gratitude did not feature," she insists.

And those who said, Someday you'll look back on this and say it's the best thing that ever happened to you—well, she remembers listening with one ear and letting that happy claptrap float out the other.

"Because I was more about hurt and revenge than gratitude. Gratitude was way too positive an emotion for me to feel," she says. "Wallowing. Now, there was something I could master."

And she did. Until that day when wallowing felt a teeny bit icky. And slightly restrictive. And not much fun.

"By the time wallowing felt thoroughly icky and extremely restrictive and absolutely no fun—I was ready to be open to a tiny bit of positive," Michele says. "I was a human opinion graph, and started edging the slider away from red/angry toward blue/happy."

And that's when gratitude got a toehold in her life.

She remembers, "I wasn't paying a ton of attention. Just, one day, there it was. Gentle glimmers of gratitude."

"I bid a cautious welcome and began counting the ways I was grateful," she says. "Just one a day to start. Then two. Then three. Then a whole slew. A slew of gratitude graced my consciousness."

She checks off her list of things appreciated: "I was grateful that I was no longer with a man who could not be faithful. I was grateful that I was no longer centering my life on someone who did not return the favor. I was grateful that I no longer had to share my finances with someone less than financially responsible. I was grateful for the one-on-one time with myself, and with my children. I was grateful for the people who came into my life, bringing love and humor and compassion. I was grateful for having had my own resilience and strength tested—and passing the test. I was grateful to know that even in the depths of my despair I was not alone. Could never be alone. Was absolutely loved. By God and the whole universe. Even by myself."

And that's when Michele stopped telling the story. Because it no longer reflected her. Or served her. Or fueled her.

"I had found the fuel of pure gratitude," she says. "The worst thing I could possibly have imagined had happened to me—and it was OK. In fact, more than OK. Because today I look back and see a marriage that I loved but that needed to end. And I see a me that needed to grow. And I see a life that needed to be lived. Lived in gratitude."

So now she does.

"And so can you," says Michele. "Even if the worst thing you could possibly imagine has happened to you. Because you are not alone. You are loved. You will pass the test. And that's something to be grateful for."

GRATITUDE PRACTICE

Try this mudra *(a yogic hand gesture) that is a way to bless yourself and remind yourself that you are protected and loved. Hold your thumb and your first two fingers together and circle your heart while you chant, "One earth, one people, and one love." Repeat as many times as you want. It reminds you that you are one with the earth and the people who love you.*

EXPERIENCE WHAT REALLY MATTERS

The hardest arithmetic to master is that which enables us to count our blessings.

—Eric Hoffer

Sometimes, people we trust are the very ones who disappoint us the most. We want to curse them and ourselves for not reading the signs, not getting it that the person was not friend, but foe.

But we can't go there. We need to look to those who teach the lesson that there are givers and then there are takers; that in trusting we should be grateful for the soul of ourselves that is open, trusting, and believes in others.

That's the good news in betrayal. We need to give thanks to the part of us who cared, and let go of those who have yet to receive that blessing. Anne and Joe Roberts *share their experience in moving on and giving thanks for lessons learned.*

As Anne Roberts remembers it, the year 2007 started with all the hope, promise, and optimism only the new beginnings of January can bring. Anne, who owns Access Elevator Supply in Emeryville, California, with her husband, Joe, was looking forward to the promise of prosperity and what lies ahead.

But by the end of the month her family's lives were shattered after they discovered that an employee they had promoted to general manager over a career of 10 years had been embezzling from the company for six of those years.

Anne was devastated. Trusts, loyalty—both were betrayed. The employee had come to them highly recommended by industry peers. She had gained their trust with her hard work, drive, talent, and initiative.

"In hindsight, we never should have given over that much control to anyone," Anne says. "This employee systematically gained our trust and took over functions of our company that would give her access to the money coming in. Of course she was the first one my husband turned to when we were trying to uncover what was going on. We later learned she had five ways she used to steal from us, and the amounts were high—very high."

She continues, "All the employees were in a state of shock. We all had been fooled. To the credit of our employees, our customers never knew what was being uncovered that year. Because the industry is small and she was well known by those calling our office, the word did get out eventually. Everyone was shocked. All the employees were a tremendous help at this time."

Due to the numerous ways the thefts were carried out, the company will never have conclusive numbers for the loss, but they estimate it was close to $350,000.

So, how does one find gratitude in this situation?

Anne is grateful for the people who helped prosecute this employee and make her accountable for her actions. And she is grateful for the lessons this experience taught her. As she learned how to peel away the anger, hurt, and betrayal and deal with only the facts, she came to the realization that "there is something very refreshing about dealing with just the known."

Reflecting on the experience, she says, "We tend to wander amongst the unknown, and that is a dangerous place to hang out. I appreciate the moment much more because I experienced how quickly things can change. I am grateful for the ability to identify what is truly important and realize that money is *never* associated with those things. Thus, I am grateful for true friends, a loving, compassionate family, and the natural beauty that surrounds us every day. Even a storm at sea is beautiful when viewed through the window of safety."

Anne has learned that gratitude is something that

cannot be imposed on others. It must be heartfelt. And, as feelings are self-generating, one usually learns gratitude through life experiences. We learn some lessons from negative events, but they can be a tremendous opportunity for growth. Anne and Joe Roberts have learned to focus with gratitude on the many blessings in their lives.

GRATITUDE PRACTICE
To truly practice gratitude, say thank you for challenging experiences, for people who have hurt or betrayed us. Send them light. Forgive yourself; it's not your fault. Count your blessings, as by blessing we are blessed. And move on.

RX FOR LIFE: GRATITUDE

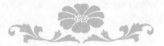

> He is a wise man who does not grieve for the
> things which he has not, but rejoices for those
> which he has.
>
> —*Epictetus*

*In times of trouble or transition, when we are feeling
down or afraid, the best medicine can be hope and gratitude. To be grateful gives us hope, and hope lets us know
that things can get better, that we can move through our
situations and get to the other side.*

*Given her story, Julie Comeau might be mired in self-
pity and weighed down by negative emotions 24/7. With
multiple medical setbacks that have left her unable to live
the life she wants, Julie might be very resentful. But she
believes instead that where there is a tiny ray of sunshine,
even just a sliver, the sun will come out again.*

In November 2005, Julie Comeau, of Fredericton, New Brunswick, was working at her job in a hospital laundry. While pulling a heavy laundry cart with a defective wheel, she heard a loud pop and screamed out in pain. She was unable to move her right leg and noticed a bulge emerging from under her rib cage on the right side. Thus began a four-year medical nightmare that included a misdiagnosis and surgery she did not need.

Today, at 39, she is waiting for her final operation after enduring a series of medical mishaps that have left her unable to walk properly and with severe nerve damage to certain parts of her body.

Julie recalls how the nightmare began. Following her accident and a meeting with her family doctor, a vascular surgeon confirmed that she had a hernia, and she was scheduled for surgery on December 15th, 2005.

"No tests were done before my surgery to confirm what my injury was. The surgeon said no tests were needed, for he was certain that my injury was a hernia," Julie says. "When I awoke, the surgeon was standing by my bedside and told me that he cut into the bulge underneath my right rib cage as far as my colon and could find no hernia at all. Then he went on to inform me, 'Wrong operation—your injury is much deeper down into your leg and I am not qualified to go down that far, so I am going to have to send you to see someone else.' "

Julie couldn't believe what she was hearing. "There I am with an operation that I did not need and the injury was still in my body," she says. "As I healed from the wrong operation I noticed that I couldn't lift my right leg without the help of my hands. The strength in the top part of my leg was gone, and this was something new. I discovered that this wrong operation must have caused muscle damage at the top part of my leg."

Unbelievably, this was Julie's third experience with medical mishaps. She now lives with permanent nerve damage and muscle spasms in the left side of her chest that often take her breath away with severe pain. She also suffers with paralysis and nerve damage to the left side of her neck and throat, as well as muscle damage to her right leg and a four-year-old injury that still has not yet been fixed.

"My leg injury has taken away my ability to walk properly, drive my car, jog, bike, or sit," Julie says. "I can't go on nature walks with my family, walk my dog, swim, dance, or just be myself. I spend most of my day lying on bags of ice to keep the swelling down and have to freeze my leg due to all the pain. After four years, we have finally found a doctor in Montreal who is going to do his best to try and help me walk again properly, but I have been told that due to all the neglect I will never be a hundred percent."

But through it all, Julie remains grateful for what she *has*. "For all that has happened to me, I know I have so much more gratitude for life than I ever did before," she says. "I now appreciate the little things: a smile, a touch, a look, just being able to tell my husband and my boys how much I love them, or being able to give them a hug and tell them how proud I am of them. Just being there in the moment with the ones you love."

Despite her many setbacks, Julie says she is grateful to be loved and supported by her husband and sons and by so many people. Along the way, she is grateful for the other angels who have come to her family's aid. Wayne and Walter Gretzky and Jason Williams of the Detroit Red Wings have joined forces with her community to help the family raise money for care.

"Sometimes I look out my window and find the tallest tree and watch a squirrel jump from branch to branch, or just the joy of watching a butterfly go from flower to flower or fly in tall grass," she says. "I appreciate how beautiful the water is when the moon hits it, or a rainbow after a hard rain. Or a bird as it sits still just for a moment, then flies away... These are just some of the things that I have more gratitude for, and just being thankful for waking up each morning and knowing God has given me one more day. For all these things I am thankful."

For Julie, the lessons come down to the simple premise to be grateful for what we have, not regret what we've lost.

"As I go through this life, no matter how tough life has been, and still is, and no matter how my injuries have consumed me—I go through life not concentrating on the things I cannot do but on the things that I can still do. And for that I am thankful."

GRATITUDE PRACTICE
Lee Brower, founder and CEO of Empowered Wealth LC, collects and gives away "gratitude rocks." He advises people to put one in their pocket, and every time they touch it take a moment to think about something they're grateful for.

PUTTING TOGETHER THE BROKEN PIECES
TO CREATE A MOSAIC OF THANKS

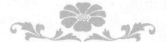

Whenever you find tears in your eyes, especially unexpected tears, it is well to pay the closest attention. They are not only telling the secret of who you are, but more often than not of the mystery of where you have come from and are summoning you to where you should go next.

—Frederick Buechner

Hardship often plays a significant role in birthing gratitude. There is a tension between wallowing in self-pity and turning that energy into tools of giving and gratitude—the whole glass-half-full concept.

When brokenness and suffering enter our lives, we have a choice whether to let it simmer and stew, depleting our sense of peace, faith, and hope for healing and love.

That is the time when we have to be purposeful about bringing fresh ideas and perspectives, along with a greater sense of possibility, in place of the weariness sinking in to our broken places. Here, we are inspired by a family who

have moved beyond their child's terminal illness to create
a shining mosaic of thankfulness and giving back.

Imagine sitting in the intensive care unit of a hospital with doctors, nurses, and support staff telling you your newborn son is not going to make it. Scott and Penni Newport have lived this moment many times in the seven years since their son Evan was born. He was diagnosed with a terminal heart disease and a variety of other complications brought about by a genetic condition called Noonan's syndrome. At his birth the Michigan couple were told, "Children like Evan usually don't live past the age of two." It is a refrain they have heard over and over and over again.

"I remember telling a nurse, 'I know Evan will probably die, but I want to thank you for helping our family in this very difficult time,' " Scott, a carpenter, says. "She wept."

But even though there has never been a moment of "normal" life since the day Evan entered their lives, the family—Scott, Penni, their son Noah, and Scott's daughter Chelsea from a first marriage—have focused not on the limitations of Evan's illness but instead on what Scott calls "the glory and gratitude we have every day."

Grateful for the significant role nurses, doctors, therapists, and all those who have helped Evan have played, Scott turned to what he knows best to express his thank-you to them. In the last seven years, he has crafted more

222

than 500 pieces of furniture—doll houses, wooden tables and benches, treasure chests, and more—which he has given to medical staff or donated to the pediatric department of Mott Children's Hospital, where Evan has spent most of his seven years. All of the items have been made from broken pieces of wood, scraps from his workshop, which he has salvaged and repurposed as beautiful gifts.

"I think all that broken stuff is a metaphor for kids like Evan, who others might think are broken, or throwaways, but they are blessings, and special gifts for us all," Scott says. "So I take what would be thrown in a dumpster and make it into an end table or a memory chest. What has been so wonderful is how sweet all the doctors and nurses have been about the gifts. Every one of them has made sure the furniture is given to a child or family it would be perfect for."

And Scott's handiwork has found its way into the White House. The George W. Bush family even invited the Newports for a visit to say thanks for a piece of furniture Scott made out of sycamore wood (which he points out can be read as "sick or more").

"The lesson I've learned from Evan and want to share with you is, in the midst of a difficult life event, don't give up," says Scott. "Don't give audience to thoughts of 'If only...' and 'I wonder if...' and 'I wish that...' Embrace joy where you find it—in the poignant, the bittersweet, and the temporary. Those moments are sometimes so subtle they flutter into our lives for just a moment, and if we're not paying attention, they're gone in the next blink."

Scott says he has learned to embrace the special moments in every day—it is one of his tools for living. When he needs reasons to be thankful, he thinks of Evan, who, he says, wakes up smiling every day. His son is tethered to a ventilator to breathe, uses signs to communicate, and has been in and out of hospice throughout his life. Yet he has defied the odds and survived every time someone told them, "This is it."

"He loves life," Scott says.

"Sometimes people ask Penni and me, 'Wouldn't it be great if you guys could go back? You know, reset your lives to a time before Evan was born?' And sometimes we hear comments like 'That's such a shame.' 'It's just not fair.' 'Do you guys ever go out just to escape?' Or the worst: 'He's going to get better, isn't he?' No, I tell them, Evan isn't going to get better. The disease he has is incurable. Every time, their faces fall. And as I break this news to them, some small part of me must accept that reality all over again myself."

He continues, "But even if I could, I wouldn't reset my life to before he was born. Sure, there are times when I wonder what that would be like. But life B.E. (before Evan) would be missing all the things Evan has given us: A higher standard to live by. More compassion for others. A rare sense of how precious life is.

Scott says he receives a blessing every day when he walks from his woodshop into the house after working. He reflects, "I know many of us wonder at times why children like Evan have to be born different. Why do they have to be broken and unrepairable? I think the answer, though not always obvious, is because they teach us things we never would have learned without them. Evan teaches us that all people matter, and that all people have worth no matter what. And for that, I give thanks every day."

GRATITUDE PRACTICE
Practice this whenever life throws you a bump.

When confronted with a situation that appears fragmented or impossible, step back, close your eyes, and envision perfection where you saw brokenness. Go to the inner place where there is no problem, and abide in the consciousness of well-being.

—*Alan Cohen*

TEN WAYS TO SAY THANKS FOR BEING THERE AND TO CULTIVATE A GRATEFUL HEART

1. Be grateful and recognize the things others have done to help you.

2. When you say "thank you" to someone it signals what you appreciate and why you appreciate it.

3. Post a "Thank you to all" on your Facebook page or your blog, or send individual e-mails to friends, family, and colleagues.

4. Send a handwritten thank-you note. These are noteworthy because so few of us take time to write and mail them.

5. Think thoughts of gratitude—two or three good things that happened today—and notice calm settle through your head, at least for a moment. It activates a part of the brain that floods the body with endorphins, or feel-good hormones.

6. Remember the ways your life has been made easier or better because of others' efforts. Be aware of and acknowledge the good things, large and small, going on around you.

7. Keep a gratitude journal or set aside time each day or evening to list the people or things you're grateful for today. The list may start out short, but will grow as you notice more of the good things around you.

8. Being grateful shakes you out of your self-absorption and helps you recognize those who've done wonderful things for you. Expressing that gratitude continues to draw those people into your sphere.

9. Remember this thought from Maya Angelou: "When you learn, teach; when you get, give."

10. Join forces to do good. If you have survived illness or loss, you may want to reach out to others to help as a way of showing gratitude for those who reached out to you.

CHAPTER TEN

PUTTING GRATITUDE INTO ACTION: GRATITUDE TOOLS

As we express our gratitude, we must never forget that the highest appreciation is not to utter words, but to live by them.

—John Fitzgerald Kennedy

Throughout this book, we have learned that in good times and in times of uncertainty alike, we can be inspired by or take solace in the hope that gratitude brings to our lives. For those of us who feel fortunate today as we consider the imprint that thankfulness has made in our lives, we look ahead with a tremendous sense of gratitude.

We've learned from the wealth of examples in these inspirational and heartwarming stories how gratitude can make a difference—and can actually change the direction of our lives. Let these stories inspire you to live with gratitude each and every day.

Just think what our world would be like if we all adopted an attitude of gratitude in every arena of our lives—at home, at the office, at the grocery store, in chance encounters with strangers.

Studies have shown that even businesses thrive and grow with a touch of thankfulness added to the product mix. In one experiment, a jewelry store owner who called and thanked each of his customers showed a 70 percent increase in purchases. By comparison, those whose customers were told about a sale showed only a 30 percent increase in purchases, and customers who were not thanked did not show an increase in buying behavior.

What we can learn from this is that just as we create an exercise plan for our health, or map out recipes for healthy eating, we need to put gratitude first—literally, and create a daily ritual for giving thanks.

A YEAR OF LIVING GREAT-FULLY: 50 WAYS TO SAY THANK YOU EVERY DAY

God gave you a gift of 86,400 seconds today. Have you used one to say "Thank you"?

—William A. Ward

Realizing that we are part of a greater whole is one of the fundamental keys to well-being. Those who accept the guidance and direction within themselves discover a force that yields joy and thankfulness.

Wanting to do something to empower herself, but more importantly pay tribute to her lifelong belief that we are here to help each other, Elida Witthoeft turned to creative service to others. In her story we see how, by following our inner wisdom and celebrating life and our role in the greater scheme of the universe, we can tap into the power of grace and gratitude every day.

In 2007, the year Elida Witthoeft turned 50, she decided to dedicate herself to "The Year of 50 Good Things." Her younger cousin had recently been diagnosed with a recurrence of breast cancer, so she decided to make the Race for the Cure her centerpiece. In early June (right before the big b-day), the Unionville, Connecticut, resident walked the race and raised more than $2,000 for breast cancer research.

That was just her first act of thankfulness. *Forty-nine to go.*

"All year, I sought things to do to add to the list," Elida, a senior news editor at ESPN, recalls.

She volunteered time at a local children's museum during Black History Month. She donated books to local Head Start students. She donated money to causes ranging from scholarships at Northwestern University (her alma mater) to Nothing but Nets, a group that buys malaria nets for sub-Saharan African families. She served as a mentor in three mentoring programs at ESPN. She threw a party for the folks at the senior center and donated a microwave oven to the center.

"When you think about it, fifty things add up to one act a week," Elida says. "By the end of the year, I was more into finding things to do than keeping track. The entire project gave very special meaning to a landmark year in my life, and I will never forget it. I was grateful I was able to donate time and money and help people in the process."

Elida's life's adage is taken from Winston Churchill, who said, "We make a living from what we get. We make a life from what we give." She also lives by the words in Luke 12:49, "To whom much is given, much is required."

"Declaring my fiftieth year 'The Year of 50 Good Things' gave me a chance to live those beliefs," she says.

Sadly, Elida's cousin lost her battle with cancer in December 2007. She was 47. "I'll never regret the time I spent on the centerpiece of the project," Elida says.

GRATITUDE PRACTICE

In her book Heart Steps: Prayers and Declarations for a Creative Life, *Julie Cameron suggests we experiment with prayers and declarations and then record for ourselves the results we observe in our life and in our consciousness. Practice repeating this to yourself every day: "I find joy in service. I open my mind and heart to the plan of service that brings the most joy to me and others. I accept my guidance and direction as they unfold within me."*

THE POWER OF CREATING A GRATITUDE DREAM BOARD—A PLACE TO BE GRATEFUL FOR ALL GOOD THINGS

Feeling grateful or appreciative of someone or something in your life actually attracts more of the things that you appreciate and value into your life.

—Christiane Northrup

"*Build it and they will come,*" "*Seeing is believing,*" and similar slogans give life to the idea that in practicing gratitude and saying thank you for what is, you create what can be.

Katie Mattson is a firm believer that you can be or do anything you want. You just need to intentionally put your beliefs out there for them to manifest. She does this as part of an annual tradition—creating a gratitude dream board. Here, she shares her tools for tapping into the hidden power of gratitude and counting your blessings ever before they happen.

* * *

Katie Mattson has a self-actualization tool she uses to visualize what she wants to achieve and what she anticipates being grateful for. At the beginning of each year, she creates a dream board and uses it to keep track of her progress, attitude, and goals for the coming 12 months. Using magazines, words, and markers, she maps out what she wants for herself that year.

Katie starts by grabbing a stack of magazines and cutting out words that resonate with her. She advises, "Want to increase your salary this year? Write down a number. Want to lose weight this year? How much? Want to fall in love? What is he/she like? Want to buy a house? What does it look like? Be as specific as possible with your dream board." Initially she purchased a standard poster board or piece of foam core and just filled it up. More recently, she purchased a sectioned frame which can be refilled each year.

Each section is used for a different area of her life. "I use phrases and photos of things I want for myself this year: attitudes, empowerment phrases, making natural easy-flowing choices, personal mantras," she says. "In one of the sections I detailed the adventures I'd like to have this year, since traveling to see new places is really important to me. In another, I detailed what I wanted for my business. In the last, what I wanted in the way of love from family, friends, and a future partner."

Katie recommends being creative. "What is wonderful about this is that each day you can get into that grateful feeling place for 'having' each one of these. From there, as they begin to manifest themselves in your life, your gratitude skyrockets and your effort begins to double."

GRATITUDE PRACTICE
Create a gratitude dream board. Be specific with your goals. When your board is complete, write the phrase "This or something better is making its way into my life right now. I trust the Universe's plan for me." Then put it up where you can see it, or where you can take it out to look at it each day. Many people prefer placing it by their bed, on their bathroom wall, or on the refrigerator.

ATTITUDES OF GRATITUDE: GRATITUDE OPENS THE DOOR TO UNITY

In ordinary life we hardly realize that we receive a great deal more than we give, and that it is only with gratitude that life becomes rich.

—Dietrich Bonhoeffer

Sometimes we don't see what is right in front of us, the saying goes. This is often true of the blessings in our lives. Here, we are reminded that we need to put intention behind creating an attitude of gratitude in our lives.

Eileen Duhne is firm in her conviction that "Gratitude is an attitude of life." She believes that being grateful is a pattern of life that has an uplifting effect. The Fairfax, California, publicist and metaphysician enthuses, "It's like a self-fulfilling jewel: the more grateful you are, the more blessings seem to come your way."

"If you can get into a mode of gratitude, it's like magic—you can change the vibration of any situation with a dose of gratitude," she says. "It's not always easy when you don't feel so great to remember to be grateful, but it's one of the fastest ways out of a funk. An attitude of gratitude will shift the polarity of a situation and will disarm others when they are met with the nonresistance that is gratitude."

Wherever you look, look for gratitude. Eileen points to her earliest teachers as helping inspire this attitude in her. "One of the first books I read that expanded my understanding of gratitude was Louise Hay's life-transforming book *You Can Heal Your Life*. In the 'Prosperity' section she recommended being joyful when you pay your bills. It was a simple yet profound exercise in bringing gratitude into all aspects of life. If you've ever been tight financially, you know how good it can feel to pay a bill. Louise said to remember to be grateful for all that we have, even the simple things like a soft bed, heat, a warm shower. I have never forgotten this recommendation and have learned that a simple act of being thankful shifts the vibration of our lives."

Eileen revels in spontaneous bursts of thankfulness. "When something fantastic happens or I escape some drama like a fender bender, I have gotten into the pattern of saying "Thank you" out loud. I acknowledge the immediate blessing. It makes the special occurrence a sacred moment in time, plus I believe the angels who help us with life appreciate the gratitude!"

She is aware of the potency of gratitude, urging everyone to look carefully at what they should be grateful for in their lives. She recommends being grateful for what you have; for the things you envision in your life; and for that which has yet to arrive but is coming your way.

Eileen believes there is always something to be grateful for. To put your life in perspective, just think of the people in Iraq, or Darfur, she says. Most of us have it pretty good; there's always someone else who has it worse off. We just need to remember to be grateful for all our blessings.

"Thinking of or writing down all the things in your life you are grateful for, from your pet to your new car and everything in between, is a good way to cure insomnia," Eileen says.

GRATITUDE PRACTICE

Keep a pen and a journal next to your bed, and before you rise every morning, make a list of all that you're grateful for, realizing that gratitude will magnetize good things and good people to you. Gratitude also helps us open our hearts for the day.

—The Law of Attraction, from The Secret

SIXTY SECONDS OF GRATITUDE PRACTICE

Margie Lapanja of Incline Village, Nevada, has this formula for tapping into gratefulness in our lives and making every day a thank-you.

"Being grateful for the gifts you have been given, love being the most resplendent of all, is the very foundation of a timeless, joyous Celebration of Life. For the love you give *and* the love you receive to thrive with freshness, stability, and magic, always count and honor your blessings and gifts. A careless rain falls on the party whose revelers are numb with the side effects of living in a fast-forward world. If you don't make the effort to protect your love light with an umbrella of gratitude, your light will dim or be extinguished."

Here are some practices she suggests:

❁   Make a promise to yourself to consciously set aside a time each day (even if it is but sixty precious seconds) to fortify your belief in the miracle of love and keep the river of your soul flowing with clear and clean waters through the practice of gratitude.

✿ Upon waking, as you lie in bed drifting through your dreams, greet the glory of the new day with a sacred declaration of the power of love. Either aloud or in silence, recite this personal celebration of rebirth, new beginnings, and possibilities inspired by an Irish prayer, or create a canticle—and a time—of your own:

I arise this day
With love in my heart,
Through the warmth of the sun,
The radiance of the moon,
Freedom of the wind,
Joy of rushing water,
Splendor of fire,
Stability of earth,
Serenity of stars, and
the wisdom of silence.
I embrace this day
Through the grace of life to guide me
And the promise of love to inspire me.

LIGHTS, CAMERA, ACTION:
AN EPIPHANY MOMENT SHINES THE
SPOTLIGHT ON THE NEED FOR CHANGE

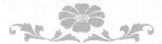

*Let us rise up and be thankful, for if we didn't
learn a lot today, at least we learned a little, and if
we didn't learn a little, at least we didn't get sick,
and if we got sick, at least we didn't die; so let us
all be thankful.*

—Buddha

*The workplace is often where our hopes and our fears
meet, where white meets black. When things aren't
exactly going harmoniously, we may find ourselves feeling
stressed out and uncertain about our futures. This can
make us fearful and sad.*

*Here, Lori Hope shares the epiphany moment when
she realized how squeezed her life at work had become.
Her decision to change was much like killing weeds. Once
she cleared away what was choking out her life, there was
room for the gift—a promise of the new.*

*As with planting seeds in a garden, Lori had to have
faith that the heavy digging and leveling was preparing*

the way for something new. From that, gratitude sprouted and grew.

Lori Hope, of Oakland, California, remembers the day as if it were yesterday. She was working with her videographer and work partner, with whom she had worked on more than 15 social documentaries.

It was the early 1990s, and as she describes herself, "I was an over-the-top intense (gosh I hate this word, but it certainly describes the old me) workaholic." Her business partner Douglas called her on it. He told her, "You're driving me crazy with your energy. It's just too much. You need to get a grip and slow down." And she remembers feeling "deeply hurt."

"I made excuses—But this is so important! I don't have a choice! Someone has to do it," she recalls.

But shortly afterward, she says, "I realized the job was killing me." To Lori, a staff producer, her life was nonstop production and she was always under the gun with deadlines for broadcasts.

Despite the fear and uncertainty, Lori remembers feeling relieved and thankful. "When I fought off the feelings of defensiveness and even a little shame, I realized my videographer was right. I felt a sense of gratitude and love wash over me. He was honest enough, and loving enough, and had enough self-respect (but also chutzpah) to say what needed to be said."

GRATITUDE PRACTICE

Lori offers this idea for expressing gratitude: "When I want to pray for someone—or keep someone in my heart, which is what I often do—I take a few deep breaths and form a picture in my mind of the individual, and focus all my attention on that image. Then I consciously send love. Saying or whispering 'I love you' using your loved one's name makes it even more powerful."

LEARNING HOW TO LIVE—AND APPRECIATE— RIGHT HERE, RIGHT NOW

We all live with the objective of being happy; our lives are all different and yet the same.

—Anne Frank

NINA'S STORY

I am grateful to the people who shared their stories in this book. They come from all walks of life with completely different stories to tell, yet they all managed to find some measure of happiness and peace in their lives.

There are so many books, institutions, professions, and pharmaceuticals devoted to helping people realign their psyches, manage their pain, and divert their energy. Throughout history, people have searched for happiness and the meaning of life. Great philosophers and writers have devoted themselves to the subject. But, Albert Camus said, "You will never be happy if you continue to search for what happiness consists of."

Yet most of us persist in believing that happiness is just around the corner—if we could just fix this, or obtain that.

Until recently, I was such a person. I thought that the way to "keep on keeping on" was to focus on dreams; I fantasized about winning my dream home in a lottery, or living a glamorous life in another city. I read books such as *Bella Tuscany: The Sweet Life in Italy* as if they were instruction manuals on how to become happy.

I also thought that the way to ward off adversity was to worry. My conversations with others seemed to center on "stress competitions"—you know, when someone describes their troubles and you outdo them with a litany of complaints? I actually thought that people would like me better if they felt sorry for me. And because I have experienced so many of the events related in this book, including losing a loved one, losing everything when my house burned to the ground, getting divorced when my children were young, and more, I always had plenty of grievances to share.

So I focused on the future, even though I knew, intellectually, and from my yoga practice, that I was supposed to live in the now. I just didn't know how to do that. I had experienced a deep state of grace—once—while lying on a hammock positively glowing from feelings of gratitude—

even toward certain people I blamed for making my life miserable—but I attributed it to being on vacation.

When I started practicing gratitude at home, I came to the realization that grateful thinking is not only the closest we can get to an *appreciation* of the here and now—it is the best way to *arrive* at the present moment. And I've discovered that if I am not in the present moment, then I am missing out on all the beauty and significance of life's joys and pleasures. It really comes down to a choice—we can choose to put our lives on hold for some indeterminate time, or we can learn to receive the gifts from our many blessings starting today. John Lennon famously said, "Life is what happens to you when you're busy making other plans," which pretty much sums it up.

What was my secret to developing an enduring feeling of contentment, self-acceptance, a deeper connection to my loved ones, and all the other affirming byproducts of increased satisfaction? I was aware of the teachings of spiritual leaders and self-help advisors, I just needed a *tool* to reprogram my superstitious thinking that something bad will happen if life is going too well. I needed to be able to replace the voice in my head that repeated, "My life sucks," when I was under stress. And that device for me is the practice of gratitude. It's really the best way I've found to relax and become mindfully present in the moment.

It wasn't something that happened to me one day; I didn't join an organization or attend any meetings. I simply reframed my thoughts. Dr. John Duffy, who writes in Chapter Five about how he consciously shifted his thinking from negative thoughts to positive ones, describes the process brilliantly.

For example, when I think about my teenage daughters (and you know how easy it is to cycle into crazy-making thoughts about teenagers!) I take a moment to give thanks for their health and for the people they turned out to be. This immediately switches my mental gearshift from fretful thinking to gratitude.

When I think about my husband, I think about what a great guy he is and how incredibly lucky I am to be married to him. Previously, I thought that if I voiced my complaints, and voiced them often, I might be able to change whatever I perceived needing changing. Then one day I realized that the life I always fantasized about is the life I am currently living. I am such a fortunate person! It didn't take a near-death experience to recognize that fact. All it took was acceptance. And noticing what was right, instead of focusing on what I thought was lacking.

Now I make it a habit to notice abundance throughout my day. When I go outside, I express gratitude for the rain, or the sunshine. When my dog is interrupting me, instead of shooing her away, I thank her for reminding me to get up from my computer to take a break. I read the news, and history books, and listen to others' stories, and feel tremendous appreciation for having been born in these times, in this country. Compare our lives to the lives of factory workers during the Industrial Revolution. Or the Irish during the potato famine. Or the victims of the Holocaust.

Tragically, there are people right here in North America struggling because they've lost their jobs, their health care benefits, or their homes. But as the stories in this book illustrate, when the worst happens it helps to be thankful for what we *do* have; this empowers us to envision a new and better future. By continuing to live in a state of conscious contentment, we may find a path to happiness and joy, and this can inspire others around us.

A study published in the *British Medical Journal* by scientists from Harvard University and UC San Diego showed that happiness spreads through social networks of family members, friends, and neighbors. Knowing someone who is happy makes you 15.3 percent more likely to be happy yourself, the study found. A happy friend of a friend increases your odds of happiness by 9.8 percent, and even your neighbor's sister's friend can give you a 5.6 percent boost.

Dr. Nicholas A. Christakis, a physician and medical sociologist at Harvard who cowrote the study, found that your emotional state is affected by the actions and choices of other people, many of whom you don't even know. Gratitude really can change the world!

GRATITUDE PRACTICE

Say thank you as many times a day as you can. It will become a daily/moment-to-moment mantra of life. Thank you for everything!

CREATE A "GRATITUDE AND GIVING CIRCLE"

Looking to incorporate gratitude as a regular part of your life? Assemble a circle of friends, family, neighbors, or colleagues for a weekly gratitude gathering. You can do this in person, or create an online community. It's a way for you to intentionally connect with one another in a special group dedicated to honoring the expression "Thank you." To learn more, check out our website, www.livinglifeasathankyou.com.

ABOUT THE AUTHORS

 NINA LESOWITZ is a gratitude practitioner who runs Spinergy Group, which represents authors and corporate clients as well as nonprofits. An award-winning marketing professional, Nina lives her life as a thank-you by acknowledging her many blessings and by giving back to the community through her volunteer work for literary organizations and schools. Born in Brooklyn, New York, Nina is has traveled extensively throughout the Far East, Europe, and Latin America. Co-author of the bestselling *The Party Girl Cookbook*, Nina lives in Piedmont, California, with her husband, Martin, and two daughters.

MARY BETH SAMMONS is a "gratitude entrepreneur" who creates new reasons each day to be thankful. An award-winning journalist and author of eight books about making a difference, including *Second Acts That Change Lives: Making a Difference in the World* (Conari Press) and *We Carry Each Other: Getting Through Life's Toughest Times*. Mary Beth has carved out a career in helping surface stories of "ordinary people doing extraordinary things," and is a frequent contributor to the *Chicago Tribune*, Beliefnet.com, and EldercareAbc.com. A cause-related marketing specialist, she helps foundations and nonprofit organizations surface their compelling stories and spread the good news. She lives with her three children in Chicago's north suburbs.